MW01168608

Elevate
YOUR HEALTH

*Inspiration and Motivation to Embrace
and Maintain a Healthy Lifestyle*

JENNIFER MELVILLE

OTHER BOOKS
BY JENNIFER MELVILLE

DEDICATION

For Mom and Dad

Mom, you are the "Queen of the Kitchen". Thank you for
nourishing me with your healthy food and love.

Dad, you have always inspired me to approach life with
a curious mind and an active body.

DISCLAIMER

The contents of this book should not be considered professional or medical advice. Always consult with your physician before beginning any exercise, fitness or nutrition program.

TABLE OF CONTENTS

INTRODUCTION

Hello! I'm so happy you decided to pick up this book. It's great that you are interested in finding ways to elevate your mindset and habits surrounding health. We already have something in common! I am constantly seeking ways to achieve my health goals; tweaking my routines, behaviours and thought patterns as I flow through the seasons of my life.

Although I am not a healthcare professional or fitness expert, health, fitness and nutrition are areas of life I am deeply passionate about. I believe strongly that taking care of our bodies is one of the keys to experiencing true happiness in life. Feeling strong and healthy from the inside out allows us to walk through our days with more vitality, positivity, energy and focus. Feeling physically balanced, healthy and strong helps cultivate a matching mental mindset.

I rely heavily on advice from industry experts when making choices about *what* foods, behaviours and activities will best serve my health goals. That being said, my personal perspective on *how* to implement their advice offers a relatable, friendly and real-life approach. Like many of you, I am busy with my family and professional obligations. I am an everyday woman who, along with my husband, is running a bustling household of two active teen boys and a pair of energetic toy poodles. I realize that maintaining a healthy lifestyle and sticking to routines can often feel like a balancing act. As an everyday woman, I am 100% human. (I don't believe in Superwoman!) I fall off the wagon at times, I reach for the unhealthy choice on occasion, and I certainly have my lazy days! More often than not though, I make choices that lead me down the path towards wellness.

The purpose of this book is not to endorse perfection or reach a final destination of optimal health! I am not here to provide specific fitness advice, or prescribe any type of diet. I am someone who has made health and wellness a priority in her life for over twenty years. I have a thirst for knowledge on the topics of fitness, nutrition and overall wellbeing, so I am constantly fine-tuning my behaviours and activities as I travel through life. Through trial and error, self-exploration and contemplation, I've learned what makes me tick. I have identified ways to inspire and motivate myself to stay on track with my goals and quest for vitality and longevity. We all connect with different approaches and mindsets. I hope some of my ideas will click with *you*!

My goal is to inspire you to take action on your health goals, reconsider some of your current thought patterns, and motivate you to keep the ball rolling.

I wasn't always the poster child for good health. During early adulthood in particular, I had a very unhealthy diet, consumed too much alcohol, and exercised sporadically at best. Slowly I came to realize that the way I was treating my body was having a detrimental impact on how much enjoyment I was getting out of life. I was in my early twenties, the prime of my life, and felt like crap! I slowly but steadily started making small changes. Over time, these small changes added up to have a huge impact on both my physical and mental health.

I have been successful at sticking to my health goals for well over twenty years, and I believe I have some useful tips to share with others who are seeking a little boost of inspiration to get them going, or keep them on track. Some of my ideas you may already be doing. Some of them may not resonate with you. Even if you walk away from this book with just one or two new tidbits of wisdom that get that fire burning in your belly, I will be satisfied! Any small step towards better health is a step in the right direction.

This book is meant to serve as a petite source of inspiration and motivation that you can refer back to time and time again. Use it to kickstart your efforts and finally set yourself on a personal journey towards health and vitality. Pull it off the bookshelf anytime you feel yourself falling off the wagon, or feel the need to hit the reset button. It's meant to serve as a great slump buster!

If you read my previous books, you will know that I love lists! I always think my books pair well with a cute little journal so you can make notes and jot down any ideas or action steps that speak to you. So, please grab that journal, along with a nice cup of tea or coffee, or a refreshing glass of water. You can tackle one chapter at a time, or read the whole piece from start to finish. Why not start with reading through the table of contents and dive into the first chapter that really sparks your interest, or addresses the issue you struggle with most?

Elevate Your Health is meant to be a zippy and inspiring read that will leave you feeling energized, motivated and literally jumping out of your chair, ready to take action! Let's dive in!

1

VISUALIZE YOUR VERSION OF ELEVATED HEALTH

What does the picture of good health look like to you? We all wish for good health, but do we even know how this looks and feels? Does it mean being able to run five miles, or contort your body into the most advanced yoga poses? Does it mean fitting into those tiny jeans from years gone by hanging in the back of your closet? Does it mean having enough energy to plough through your workday, with a bit left in the tank when you get home? Does it mean having perfect blood work and full mobility?

The definition of good or better health will look different to each and every one of us. We all have unique bodies with varying life circumstances. We are all starting at a different base level. Working towards the goal of elevating your health involves creating a customized vision of good health, defined specifically by you! Your aspirations, goals and plans will ultimately be crafted from this image of ideal health you carry in your heart and head.

Do you have a clear vision of what the best, healthiest version of you looks like? I think this is an important starting point for everybody, because before we can make a list of behaviours and actions steps, we need to know what direction we are heading. Before we can map our trajectory, we need to identify our destination (hint: the destination is a moving target).

Identify Your Why's

Identify your "why's". This is a common piece of advice among fitness and nutrition experts. In order to stick to your health goals, you need to identify *why* you want to change and improve your lifestyle. You need to identify the desire burning inside you, so you can then act in a manner that will fan its flames. Have you asked yourself why you picked up this book? Have you done some soul searching and identified the reason you would like to embrace and maintain a healthier lifestyle?

Are you on a quest to look your very best on your wedding day? Are you hoping to rock the beach in your swimsuit this summer? I will certainly admit to identifying with these "why's", but I encourage you to view your health in both present and distant terms, instead of focusing on one special day or upcoming event. I like to break my thinking and my "why's" down into short term (present day) and long term (the rest of my life) categories.

Adopt a Present-Day Mindset

In terms of living in the present, think about how you want to feel *today! Today* is the one thing that is certain. Don't you want *today* to be the very best that it can be? Would you like to feel amazing and bursting with energy *today*? Would you like to feel well-nourished and satiated *today*, fueled by food that feeds your soul and the intricate systems of your body? With a "why" of feeling healthy, vital, energetic, strong and balanced *today*, you can approach each tiny daily decision with this top of mind. What breakfast will make me feel great *today*? What movement and activity would best suit how my body feels *today*? How can I best serve my sense of wellness and happiness *today*?

Operating with a present-day mindset definitely helps me approach each small decision with a clear focus. It helps me choose to go for a hike on a Sunday afternoon, even if it's raining and I'm feeling a bit lazy. It helps me choose the side salad instead of the French fries! Even though they are all small choices, they certainly add up in the big picture of life.

Gaze Into the Far Distant Future

Your wedding might be in nine months, or summer is still six months away. These could be considered long-term "why's", but I encourage you to look much further down the line. I've noticed that the older I get, the more I am inclined to look beyond the horizon. I'm in my mid-forties, so I am starting to observe the aging of my parents' generation. It starts to hit close to home when you notice people in your life declining as they age. It is interesting to make note of those who suffer health problems, and those who seem to glide through their golden years with vitality, energy, good health and positivity. It is the latter group that inspires me. That's who I want to be when I grow old!

I realize that many health issues are outside of our control. Some people are dealt poor cards, for which there appears to be no rhyme or reason. On the other hand, the lifestyle choices we make throughout our lives can stack the odds in our favor. I'm not a gambler by nature, but in this case, I'm going to bet on exercising, eating nutritiously and reducing my stress levels as much as possible. It feels like a winning combination that not only makes me feel good *today*, but will hopefully serve me well in the long term.

I encourage you to really sit back and contemplate how you would define your "why". Take the time to actually write it down. (I really recommend keeping a wellness journal where you can store inspiring and motivating tidbits for later use.) My personal "why" is to be able to enjoy the adventure and beauty that life has to offer by feeling my very best today. It is also to adopt habits and behaviours whose benefits will extend beyond today, to the many tomorrows that are hopefully in my future. I want to age with vitality and grace!

Identify Role Models That Inspire You

If you read the dedication page at the beginning of this book, you will know that I in part dedicated it to my dad. He has been inspiring me my entire life, but at the age of eighty-three, I look up to him more than ever. He lives his life with curiosity, energy and gusto, and I believe his philosophy to keep moving is one of the key secrets to his youthful body and mind. Yes, he has his aches and pains, and isn't as strong as his thirty-year-old self, but he is the heathiest version of his current self. He goes to the gym three days a week, he cycles, he hikes, he works on his cars and he guzzles the most nutrient-packed smoothies you could imagine. (I'm not sure how appetizing they are, but they sure are healthy!) I guess I have been both subconsciously and consciously soaking in his influence my entire life, and I feel fortunate to have had such a positive role model to look up to.

I always enjoy getting a newsy hometown update from my mom, as she is still in contact with many people who had a positive influence on me growing up. I was not at all surprised to hear that my old Girl Guide leader, who is now in her nineties, baked and delivered a whopping forty-six dozen Christmas cookies this past holiday season. Just as I would have expected, she is still thriving and going strong. Even as a young child, I recognized and admired that she was someone who embraced a healthy way of living. It's obvious that her lifelong dedication to a healthy lifestyle is paying off.

Do you have someone in your life that is a shining example of living and aging well? Why not make them your muse? Look to them for inspiration and marvel at the possibility of living with vitality, energy and good health well into your seventies, eighties and beyond! You don't even need to know someone in real life to be inspired by their lifestyle. I recommend reading *The Blue Zones: Lessons for Living Longer from People Who've Lived the Longest* by Dan Buettner. The book is full of interesting statistics and evidence, but what I enjoyed most were the personal stories and profiles of the people. It really solidified my desire to behave in ways today that will increase my odds of not just a long life, but one of health and enjoyment.

Make a List of Quick-Hit Inspiration

In addition to recording my "why" statement in my journal, I maintain a quick-hit list of words that inspire me. When all pulled together, they capture perfectly my definition of health and vitality. This can be a fun exercise that can serve as a spark to get some motivation bubbling inside you.

I suggest grabbing your journal and writing down a list of words that speak to you and define your image of health and wellness. To get you started, I'll share some of mine. These words resonate with me and represent all the qualities I wish to embody and exude!

- Glowing
- Fit
- Strong
- Powerful
- Energetic
- Motivated
- Inspired
- Grounded
- Balanced
- Sturdy
- Vigorous
- Thriving
- Active
- Muscular
- Peppy
- Spunky
- Dedicated
- Persistent
- Graceful
- Vibrant
- Poised
- Passionate
- Powerful

This list is great to keep on hand and refer to now and then, especially when you are feeling frustrated or discouraged. Reminding yourself of all these delicious words that you aspire to be can often be enough to turn around a mood or save you from a weak moment.

Collect Visual Inspiration

Although I definitely identify more with the written word, I also draw on visuals now and then to inspire and motivate me. If you are more of a visual person, you may find that creating a good old-fashioned vision board (physical or virtual) is an effective approach that can keep you on track with your goals. I do this now and then using Pinterest.

For instance, in March of 2020 I was feeling particularly out of balance. I felt strong, but tight and inflexible.

My focus that month was to commit to a four-week yin yoga program in an effort to improve my flexibility. I also took up barre (a form of exercise that blends ballet, yoga and Pilates) as I was looking to improve my posture and balance and learn to move with more fluidity and grace. I created a Pinterest board with inspiring quotes about balance, flexibility and patience. It included images of some of the yoga poses I was working on, as well as pretty pictures and colors that represented grace and elegance in my mind. These included photos of ballerinas, delicate flowers and soft, feminine color palettes. As the month rolled along, I would reach for this Pinterest board during cozy downtime, adding new images and scrolling those on file. It served as an encouraging and inspiring space to visit, and kept my goals top of mind during that month.

Elevating Actions and Inspiration

- If you are looking to make meaningful and lasting changes to improve the state of your health, it is important to identify your "why's". Take the time to identify the driving force behind your desire to elevate your health. Write down your reasons and motivations in a journal. Refer back to your notes when you feel discouraged or hopeless. Your own words and vision will serve as powerful inspiration to keep you on track, or get you back in the saddle.

- Adopt a present-day mindset when considering the motivation behind your desire to change. As you go through your day, ask yourself how each small decision you face will affect your wellbeing in that moment. How will your stomach feel in five minutes if you gobble down the bag of chips? How will your body feel if you choose to attend the thirty-minute yoga class? How will your body feel if you choose to skip the class and binge watch Netflix instead (likely while eating the chips)?

- Think long-term and visualize yourself in ten, twenty or thirty years. What does longevity and healthy aging look like to you? What types of activities do you want to be able to participate in throughout your life?

- Identify positive role models that inspire and motivate you. Their enthusiasm can be infectious! Learn from their example. Ask them questions about their approach to fitness, nutrition, mindset, aging…etc. Allow a little bit of their zest and magic to rub off on you!

- Create some inspirational content for your wellness journal. Try coming up with a list of ten (or more) words that capture your definition of an elevated state of health. Add to the list regularly as you identify with new ideas and goals.

- Create a mood board or Pinterest board full of images that embody the vision you have for yourself. Instead of mindlessly scrolling social media during downtime, pull up your board and really soak in the vibe and energy that you created for yourself. Use it as a tool to keep your vision of health fresh and top of mind.

2

DROP THE MONDAY MINDSET

How many times have you been inspired to start a new fitness routine or nutrition plan, only to tell yourself, "I'll start that on Monday"? While waiting for Monday to roll around, you cram in as much forbidden food and lazy lounging as possible, knowing such indulgences will soon be out of reach under your new plan. It's really a self-destructive form of procrastination that often not only delays you from reaching your goals, but can sideline them completely.

By the time Monday finally arrives, that spark of enthusiasm that was bubbling inside you just a few short days ago may have short-circuited. You no longer feel motivated to follow through with your grand plans, and find yourself continuing to wallow in your unhealthy habits. A few days later, you once again get a jolt of motivation, but sabotage yourself once more with the same old "Monday mindset". It's a vicious and agonizing cycle that frequently leads you on a path to nowhere.

What is it about human nature that makes us crave order, straight lines and clean starts? I am a professional accountant by trade, and I assure you there is no one who loves order and symmetry more than I do. It definitely feels instinctual to want to start at the beginning, whether it is an imaginary, self-imposed start line or not.

Yes, most fitness program calendars seem to start on a Monday. We clearly associate setting big goals and resolutions with the turn of the calendar to the new week, month or year. Perhaps human nature doesn't just crave order, but is drawn to seek any excuse to procrastinate as well! Maybe it is change we are afraid of and subconsciously avoiding. I think the Monday mindset is really just our way of delaying action and perceived discomfort so we can sit in the coziness and security of our current situation just a teeny bit longer. What's a few more days of unhealthy eating and lack of exercise in the grand scheme of things? While this might be true, if viewed as a one-time event on its own, we all know the Monday mindset is often a habit we play on repeat.

Challenge Your Reasoning

If you catch yourself falling into the Monday mindset trap, I encourage you to sit back and reflect. Can you take a moment to dig a little deeper into your psyche and determine what part of you wants to delay your health goals for just a few more days or months? Do you have a bit of "fun" planned in the near future, and you think healthy lifestyle changes will cramp your style? Let's say you have a girls' night on the agenda for Saturday evening. You don't want to be weighed down with thoughts of how your night out with friends, food and drinks is going to fit into your new eating plan. It just feels easier to deal with it on Monday and go from there.

Why not rethink the scenario? You can choose to start making healthier food choices this very moment, on a regular, uneventful Thursday. When Saturday rolls around, you can still make healthy food choices all day long, knowing that you will indulge in a few treats that evening. This scenario, even with the Saturday night goodies, still has you further ahead than if you put your goals on the back burner until Monday.

The holidays are coming up, and you think it would be best to just wait until the New Year to start your fresh fitness and healthy eating plan. You think to yourself, "There is no point starting my plan in mid-November with such a busy schedule of events overflowing with temptation."

I urge you to rethink this line of reasoning. The holiday season is actually a wonderful time to start a regimen of healthy habits. There is so much stress associated with this time of year, your body needs nourishing self-care during this time more than ever! Again, even if you slip up during the holidays and over-indulge on occasion, you will still be further ahead in attaining better health if you are doing your best most days. Exercising and eating well during the holidays will give you more energy, balance and a sense of wellbeing, allowing you to enjoy the season with your loved ones even more.

No day is off limits to cross the start line! Why not take an invigorating family walk on Christmas day to kickstart your new fitness goals? Any day of the week, month or year is a perfect time to celebrate and participate in steps towards good health.

Customize Your Plan

If you are truly one of those people who just can't stand starting day one of your six week fitness program on a Wednesday, when the pre-printed calendar clearly begins on Monday, just take a deep breath. I can relate! Go ahead and rewrite the plan and print yourself a fresh copy! I have done this many times and tweaked workout plans to specifically fit into my own calendar. You get to make the rules, so take charge and adjust as required. The accountant in me loves ticking boxes off my calendar when the workout is complete, so I just make sure the calendar fits my life. I have found that the act of "making it my own" encourages me to be more committed and invested in my plans.

If you still firmly feel the need to start that six week program on Monday, then at least get busy in the days leading up to the start of the week. Devise a simple warm-up plan and get yourself moving; anything you need to do to squash the dreaded Monday mindset!

Ride the Wave of Enthusiasm

Don't let that initial wave of enthusiasm to start a journey towards better health pass you by and head to shore without you riding on its crest. If you are feeling inspired while reading this book, capitalize on those tingly feelings of positivity and possibility whizzing around inside you. This very moment is when you should take that first step towards healthier habits.

I'm going to borrow Nike's timeless slogan here and say, "Just Do It!". I don't think I even own one piece of Nike clothing, but I use this statement as a form of self-talk all the time, and I find it to be very effective. Don't wait until tomorrow! Start in this very moment. Even if you ate an unhealthy lunch, you don't have to write off the day. Start making better choices with your next snack or at dinner time. Even if the series of fitness classes you signed up for starts in two days, take some time to move your body today by doing a stretching routine or going for a walk or run. Have you ever regretted taking action in the moment towards a personal goal? Have you ever regretted the choice to get up from the couch and press play on the workout? Have you ever regretted choosing the hearty, vibrant and nourishing Buddha bowl over the greasy burger?

Elevating Actions and Inspiration

- Recognize those moments when you find yourself falling into the trap of the Monday mindset.

- Challenge your desire to delay your start date. Dig a bit deeper and ask yourself why you want to put off adopting healthier habits any longer. Be honest with yourself! Push through the urge to wait and find at least one small step you can take today to move towards your goals.

- If you are following a pre-made plan that doesn't quite match your schedule and calendar, make the necessary adjustments to customize it to suit you. You are the boss and get to make all the rules! At the end of the day, the only person you are reporting to is yourself.

- Embrace those moments in time where you find yourself feeling electrically inspired and motivated. Jump at the opportunity to ride the wave of your own enthusiasm.

- Develop strategies to inspire yourself. "Just do it" is still my favorite expression to get myself moving on anything I find myself avoiding (big or small). Seek out a phrase or mantra that resonates with you and keep it in your back pocket for moments of weakness.

3

GET EDUCATED

The wellness industry is a booming business, and there is no shortage of information out there on the topics of health, fitness and nutrition. It's a bewildering and overwhelming path to navigate, with conflicting and confusing information coming at us from all directions.

I encourage you to just sit back, take a deep breath and look beyond the headlines. Dig a bit deeper than what you are being served by the media outlets. Knowledge is power, and taking the time to educate yourself on health topics will give you the information, confidence and inspiration you need to make healthy, informed decisions for yourself.

Start With the Basics

I've had an interest in nutrition and food science ever since I was a little girl, whether I realized it at the time or not. As a home economics teacher, my mother studied nutrition at university, so it was a topic that was prevalent and frequently discussed in our home. I remember scrutinizing the black and white images in her old textbooks, making a mental note that scurvy was not something I was interested in developing. (Visions of bleeding gums and missing teeth had me highly motivated to gobble up the vitamin C rich foods on my plate!) *Canada's Food Guide* had a steady presence on our refrigerator door, and Mom's meals were always well-rounded and heavy on the veggies. My parents tended a vegetable garden during the summer months, and I had my own little patch were I proudly grew a row of leaf lettuce and a few radishes and carrots. Although I definitely strayed from these wholesome eating values when I left my mother's nest and headed to university, this unhealthy period of my life didn't last long. In my mid-twenties I was drawn back to those deeply planted roots from my upbringing.

You don't need a degree in nutrition to learn how to eat for good health! It is, however, worth educating yourself on the topic. I'm certainly not in a position to recommend any one way of eating or push any of the latest and greatest diets. I'm just suggesting that you take a keen interest in the topic of food and nutrition so you can make educated decisions for yourself.

Reading a few general nutrition books, or even taking an online course or two, is a great way to learn the basics. At a minimum, it's important to be aware of the various macronutrients, vitamins and minerals our body needs, what roles they play, and what foods offer good sources. It is also useful to learn about appropriate portion sizes and the basic caloric needs for each member of your family. (As a mother of two active teens boys, I consider this information in order to ensure they are eating enough nutritious food to fuel their growth and development.)

Develop a Thirst for Deeper Knowledge

Learning about nutrition is a personal passion of mine, so I decided to dive a little deeper into the topic. Two years ago I completed a certificate in plant-based nutrition offered through e-Cornell. I was keenly interested in learning more about the science behind plant-based eating, instead of relying on shallow and superficial articles on the news and in magazines.

As I mentioned above, I'm not here to recommend any one way of eating. I'm personally drawn to a vegan diet because I was never a lover of animal products to begin with. As a child, I shed many tears at the dinner table because I simply didn't have the stomach to clear the meat products off my plate. (My term for roast beef was roast cow, which didn't have an appetizing ring to it at the age of five.) I was so happy when I turned twelve and we finally got a dog, something I had been dreaming about forever. That little beagle gobbled up everything I stealthily slipped under the table. (I feel guilty about it now, because I know it wasn't healthy for him to be eating table scraps!)

Eating a diet free of animal products just feels like "coming home" to me. It is what I naturally crave. What feels right for you may look very different. We each have to choose the path to wellness that works for our individual bodies, values and lifestyles.

Wanting to convert to full plant-based eating, I needed to ensure I was getting adequate nutrition from my diet, since I was eliminating two significant groups of food (meat and dairy). The courses I took through e-Cornell were helpful in teaching me how to design an eating plan that covered all the bases. I feel like I can now rest easy that I am not depriving myself of anything crucial by eating in this manner.

Taking things a step further and diving into the topic of nutrition is very motivating when it comes to sticking to your goals. I actually find myself inspired by the science of it all. I think a lot of people walk around with what I refer to as the "Chocolate Easter Bunny Mindset". I know I have been guilty of this in the past! We view our bodies as just a solid (or hollow) hunk of "stuff" and don't consider all the microscopic reactions and interactions going on inside. When you learn the effects of food at the cellular level, it makes you stop and think twice before biting into that donut. What exactly happens to your liver when it receives a sudden rush of sugar? What chemical conditions allow cancer cells to flourish and multiply? A strong understanding of what makes your body tick can certainly lead to better decision making.

Online nutrition courses are widely available, so if this is something that interests you, I encourage you to investigate some options. Since I personally have experience with e-Cornell, I can definitely recommend their programs. They are engaging, well-run and of high quality. If plant-based eating isn't really your thing, they do offer a more general certificate program called *Nutrition and Healthy Living*. I might drop this on my bucket list for the future.

Adopt a Critical Mind

One important take-away I gained from my e-Cornell courses was the ability to think more critically. When I hear a health claim that appears too good to be true, I immediately tune into my Spidey-senses. I approach information with a healthy dose of skepticism, and I encourage you to do the same. Next time you come across a piece of information, challenge yourself to dig a little deeper and do a bit more research. We covered an entire unit on reading the fine print behind scientific studies. It's always worth making note of who funded a study. Is it a coincidence that the results fall in favour of a product the funding company conveniently sells? I'm not suggesting that studies are inaccurate. I do, however, approach information with a bit more skepticism these days. I make sure to gather all the data I can and consider opposing perspectives before passing judgement.

Seek Expert Advice

The fitness industry is another domain where information overload is the norm. I'm not one to get wrapped up in the latest and greatest fat-burning craze. I tend to skim over most of what is out there and just stick to a basic common sense approach. I move my body daily and participate in activities and exercises that bring me joy and a sense of strength and wellness.

That being said, I believe that seeking advice from a fitness professional is important, especially when first starting out. When it comes to exercising, no matter what activity you might be participating in, using proper form and technique should be your top priority. It is amazing what an impact a little adjustment or tweak can have on not only performance, but on injury prevention.

I have been lifting weights for over two decades. When I first started, I tapped into the services a personal trainer at the gym I was attending at the time. I learned valuable information from her on how to get the most out of my workouts using a safe approach. I can't stress this point enough; safety first!

These days, all my weightlifting is done in the cozy comfort of my little basement home gym. I usually follow along with *Beachbody* videos, and their trainers are constantly pointing out tips on how to use proper technique. I installed a full-length mirror in my workout space, not as an act of vanity, but to provide a tool to keep an eye on my posture and form.

If you are starting an activity for the first time, ask for help from an experienced professional. It often takes a trained eye to see nuances that are not obvious to the rest of us. I even purchase all my running shoes from a local specialty store for this reason. Their trained staff only recommend a shoe once they have properly measured both my feet and analysed my walking and running gait. I've been running for years injury free, and I'm certain having expertly fitted footwear has contributed to this fact.

Elevating Actions and Inspiration

- With an overwhelming amount of information available on the topics of wellness, fitness and nutrition, it is wise to get educated on these subjects. You are the only one who can take control of your lifestyle decisions. Having a solid understanding of the basics will help you wade through the mass content, and pull out what feels relevant to your situation and lifestyle.

- More detailed and in-depth courses on the topic of nutrition offer an opportunity to power yourself with knowledge. Understanding the science behind nutrition can be both empowering and inspiring. This knowledge can be a key tool in keeping you on track with your health and wellness goals. (Graphic visuals of clogged arteries and diseased livers can be very motivating tools indeed!)

- Approach the diet, food, fitness and wellness industry with a critical mind. Adopting an inquisitive yet skeptical mindset will allow you to review all the facts before passing judgement.
- Consider enlisting the help of a professional fitness instructor if you are just starting out with a new program or activity. Learning to perform exercises with proper form will elevate your workouts and reduce the risk of injury.

4

PENCIL YOURSELF IN

If you had a really important appointment to attend, you would be certain to write it down in your agenda. You might even set a reminder notification on your phone for an added layer of assurance so as not to forget. What if you viewed the appointments you booked with *yourself* as top on your priority list? Why not consider your morning walk and meditation session as just as crucial to your day as the dentist appointment, your daughter's baseball game or the sales meeting?

Since you are reading this book, I'm guessing you share in my desire to make health a priority in your life. Ensuring your body gets enough regular physical activity is probably on your list of goals. It's certainly on mine, and as a result, I look for ways to make sure I fit it in most days.

Make Time

Life is busy, and most of us are trying to cram too much into our schedules as it is. I know that for many, the thought of adding one more "to do" item to their endless list feels insurmountable. "I just don't have the time to exercise", is an all too common excuse. It's easy to see why people feel this way. Our world seems to be running in overdrive, and so many people are scrambling to keep up. I do, however, argue that there are many "time wasters" that we are all guilty of engaging in.

If you feel like your days are flying by and you aren't getting anything accomplished, I suggest you perform a time audit. (I warned you that I am an accountant. Please hear me out!) I think there is often a large discrepancy between what we *think* we are spending our time on, and what we are *actually* spending our time on. Taking a day or two and to keep track of your activities might highlight some spare time in your schedule that you could put to better use.

What if you added up all these snippets of time-wasting activities in your life? Might you be able to spare thirty minutes after all to take a walk, go for a run, or hit play on a workout video? Be honest with yourself. Could you "make time" for exercise by giving up something else? Would you even miss that "something else" that is sucking up so much of your day? How much time do you spend mindlessly scrolling social media or the news websites? If you aren't sure and are curious, you can set your phone up to track your activity. The results might shock you. (They were certainly eye-opening for me!) Could the time you are frittering away on Instagram be put towards a healthier cause? What are you doing during your lunch hour at work? Could you grab your sandwich and take a walk instead of eating at your desk?

Have a Plan

One technique that has always worked for me is having a plan and actually writing it down. I guess it's not rocket science, but it's funny how we often tend to omit some of the most important "to do" items on our lists. We prioritize the needs and commitments relating to other people in our lives, but fail to pencil ourselves in at the top of the list.

Whatever form of personal organizer you use, I encourage you to tap into its potential for keeping you on track. I maintain a daily planner in paper format. (I'm old-school that way.) It's one I actually created myself with a pretty three ring binder and daily planning worksheets I custom-designed. They aren't fancy, but I wanted to ensure my planner included a specific section for health and wellness activities.

I usually sit down on Sunday afternoon and look at our family's schedule for the week ahead, as well as the upcoming weather forecast. (Since I run, my workouts can be influenced by the weather.) I then decide what my workout schedule will look like for the week and fill in my daily planning sheets accordingly. If I know I'm going to be out late Monday night for soccer practice, I might decide that Tuesday will be my day off. If they are forecasting a heavy snowfall on Thursday, I'll make sure to get my run in on Wednesday instead. I'm always sure to record both my workout plans and my daily meditation goal. That meditation goal is the one I struggle with the most! Physically writing it down on my daily to do list definitely means it gets accomplished more often than not.

By having a well-thought out plan for the week, you set yourself up for success. You enter your week with an organized mindset and a can-do attitude. Instead of flying by the seat of your pants, and squeezing in a walk or workout if you have time, you *make* time. You *schedule* time. Sure, even the best of plans can fall apart. Kids get sick, work gets crazy, life happens! The key is to follow your plan of action most of the time and to be as consistent as possible. Writing it down definitely helps in this regard.

Consider The Magic of Mornings

I am naturally a morning person. As a child, I was always the first one up on weekends. I loved tip toeing through the quiet house, grabbing myself a bowl of cereal, and settling in on the couch for my greatly anticipated line up of Saturday morning cartoons. This was in the eighties, back before the twenty four hour non-stop viewing options available today. I was usually up so early I had to wait for the station to turn on. Does anyone else remember staring at a fuzzy screen and counting down the minutes for the playing of the national anthem? (In my case it was O

Canada!) Although my teen years saw me sleeping in past noon, I rekindled my habit of rising with the birds in early adulthood.

I had just started my career working at an accounting firm, and was feeling frustrated with the sudden lack of free time I was accustomed to. We worked long hours, so my days felt pinched. I was trying to maintain an active lifestyle, but my efforts were inconsistent at best. I had a gym membership at the time, with the best intentions to hit an aerobics class after work. The overtime hours I was clocking, as well as the significant amount of travel in my schedule, were really hampering my efforts to show up for those classes. In addition, I was taking correspondence courses because I was studying for my CPA designation. If I wasn't working at night, I usually had to crack open my textbooks. Sticking to a consistent fitness routine felt like an uphill battle (and all this was before I even had kids)!

Frustrated with my failing efforts, I finally decided to take a hard look at my schedule and devise a plan that would set me up for success. I realized that my evening schedule was often out of my control. If I was working under a deadline, (which is frequent in the accounting field) I couldn't reliably commit to fitting in exercise after work.

My boyfriend (now husband) was meeting with a workout buddy at the gym *before* work. When he suggested I follow his lead, I initially balked at the idea. My immediate reaction was, "Absolutely *no way!* I need every second of sleep before that alarm starts screeching. I'm just *not* a morning person!"

I quickly realized that I was telling myself a story that wasn't necessarily true. (These "stories" we love to spin are the source of so much self-sabotage!) In fact, underneath it all, I *was* a morning person. I had been an early riser for the better part of my life. Nasty habits I adopted in my late teens and early adulthood (poor eating, excessive alcohol consumption, partying, late bedtimes) were the real reason I was no longer my chipper morning self. Besides, if my boyfriend could do it, why not me?

I begrudgingly admitted that I could probably set my alarm an hour earlier. The first few weeks were a hard adjustment, but once it became a habit, I found myself bounding out of bed in the morning. I made new friends at the gym, and even started running with a couple of them. I found I had more energy at work, and it took the pressure and guilt off my evenings. As another plus, embracing the magic of mornings forced me to rethink a number of my other lifestyle choices that were hampering my ability to rise with the sun (or before). I started eating better, quit drinking alcohol and set myself a firm bedtime. That one positive action of exercising in the morning had an elevating domino effect on my overall wellbeing. This was over twenty years ago, and I've never looked back.

If you are someone who is struggling to fit in consistent exercise, I encourage you to consider the magic the morning has to offer. It's easy to get caught up in the whirlwind of a day and have your plans sidelined by events that are out of your control. Fitting in your "me time" before the hustle and bustle of the day begins helps ensure that it gets crossed off your list. It also just feels good to start your day with self-care and taking part in an activity that is all about you! I have found getting my heart pumping each morning allows me to face each day with more energy, focus and clarity of mind.

If the thought of crawling out of bed an hour early makes you want to cry, start small! Try an extra fifteen minutes early for the first little while to let your body adjust to the new regimen. This would give you time to do some stretching, or squeeze in a quick walk. As a side note, be sure to leave your phone on the charger! Checking your email or social media first thing is a sure fire way to allow that extra time to evaporate. Make sure you use it wisely.

Once you are comfortable with the idea of setting an earlier alarm, you could then ease yourself into thirty minutes early (and eventually an hour). You can actually get a good workout done in thirty minutes or less! I run my 5K in under thirty minutes. I have done many online work-outs that offered amazing results in under half an hour!

As time goes on, you might just find yourself craving those early morning hours of tranquility and peace when the rest of the household is still sleeping. It's not uncommon for both my husband and I to be up at 5:00 a.m. most days! It really is a magical time of the day that offers an opportunity to focus on elevating actions that you can carry with you throughout your day.

The morning is a prime time to meditate. My husband (who is much more consistent with his practice than I am) swears by it. Crossing it off his list first thing in the morning ensures it gets done. He has a very hectic, fast-paced job and he feels that meditating before work allows him to have better focus and interact more positively with colleagues and clients.

Mornings offer a great opportunity to give your body a boost of nutrition. My husband starts each day with a smoothie that is jam packed with goodness. Dr. Michael Greger, one of my favorite plant-based authors, wrote a book called *How Not to Die: Discover the Foods Scientifically Proven to Prevent and Reverse Disease*. (I'll admit the title is a bit morbid, but it's chock full of intriguing information!) In it he includes a checklist of his recommended "Daily Dozen". According to Dr. Greger, we should all strive to fit this list of items into our daily routine for optimal health and longevity. My husband keeps a copy of this checklist posted on the inside of a kitchen cupboard. He challenges himself each morning to see how many items from Dr. Greger's list he can fit in his smoothie! This little game he plays with himself is a perfect way to kick off his eating habits for the day.

Even on my days off, when I'm taking a break from fitness, I'm still up with the birds (sometimes before). Don't let yourself miss out on magical mornings!

Be Flexible, Patient and Kind

I realize mornings won't work for everyone's schedule. If you work shifts, for example, you will have to be more creative and flexible with your schedule. Sometimes we hit seasons of life where old schedules and ways of doing things just don't fit with our new reality. In these situations I like to step back, catch my breath, and get creative with my approach to maintaining healthy habits.

When I was a new mom enduring sleepless nights, morning workouts were not an option! My boys were born seventeen months apart, so I essentially had two needy babies to tend to. During this period of my life, I was a sleep-deprived zombie. My husband once found me passed out on the floor in our hallway. Apparently I fell asleep on my way to our son's bedroom!

While I still exercised during this time, I had to seek out creative opportunities to fit it in. I also had to cut myself some slack. If you are a new mom, I encourage you to be patient and kind with yourself. Learn to recognize what your body needs. Some days it might be physical activity, some days it might be a nap!

I walked *a lot* with my little ones in tow during those early years. I know my boys enjoyed the fresh air, but from a purely selfish perspective, those walks helped maintain my sanity. I used to lift weights with the baby in an exersaucer and the toddler occupied with an activity. It wasn't perfect, and there were many interruptions, but I felt better and stronger for doing it. I also fit in my runs in the evenings and weekends when my husband was home from work. Again, it wasn't ideal, but I did make it work. Despite my erratic schedule and energy levels, I took the time to look at the week ahead and pencil in when and where I could fit in my exercise. Having a plan on paper gave me peace of mind and a solid goal to stick to.

Elevating Actions and Inspiration

- Put yourself and your health at the top of your list of priorities.
- If you feel pinched for time, challenge yourself to rethink your current schedule. Take a closer look at what activities in your life you are currently spending time on. Chances are you will be able to find at least thirty minutes in there somewhere!
- Consider tracking your social media and web-browsing use on your phone. The results might surprise you and unlock an opportunity to make better use of this time with health-focused activities. A great way to get your social media fix is to listen to podcasts *while* you exercise. Win-win!
- Take the time each week to create a plan for yourself around your health goals. Consider all those factors in your schedule that could have an impact on your plan and work around them.

- Physically write down your plan in your calendar or agenda. Pencil in your workouts, walks, fitness classes, meditation sessions…etc.

- Consider the possibility of exercising first thing in the morning. Not only is it a great way to start your day, but it helps ensure you fit in priority actions on your to do list. Your health goals and plans won't get sidelined by a busy day or unexpected challenges that come up.

- If you are in a situation where maintaining a regular exercise schedule feels impossible, don't give up. Take it day by day and find flexible and creative solutions that will allow you to achieve your goals.

5

DITCH THE ALL-OR-NOTHING ATTITUDE

How many times have you found yourself in a situation where an unexpected roadblock derails your grand plans towards a life of better health? How have you faced such a challenge in the past? Have you adopted an all-or-nothing attitude and thrown up your hands in defeat?

Let's say it's been three months since you embarked on your wellness journey and you are feeling fabulous! Not only have you dropped a few pounds, but you have a sense of renewed energy and enthusiasm that you haven't felt since you were a child! You've been a faithful attendee at your bi-weekly yoga classes, and have stuck to your three-days-a-week running schedule. Not only that, you've been working hard in the kitchen. You've really upped your game in the nutrition department, opting for a delicious morning smoothie and oats instead of the sugary muffin and coffee combo you were accustomed to. You've been packing healthy lunches most days instead of hitting the fast-food joints with co-workers. Meal planning has become part of your life, so you feel in control when you arrive home famished at the end of your workday. You feel like you are at the top of your game...until everything comes crashing down in one instant.

During your morning run, you misjudged your step and tripped off the edge of the sidewalk, twisting your ankle in the process. The sharp zap of pain had a foreboding feeling to it! A trip to your doctor reveals nothing is broken, but your strained tendons and ligaments took a beating. She firmly tells you to go home, ice your foot and stay off it for a few days. She warns you it could be weeks (or more!) until things have healed properly and you can return to your normal activities. You hobble home, deflated and discouraged.

What happens next is critical. Yes, you have hit a major obstacle. Yes, it feels like all of your schedules, plans and goals have been completely derailed. However, it is no time to throw in the towel, order an extra-large pizza with double cheese and flop on the couch for the next four weeks, allowing all your hard earned efforts to evaporate.

I have been in this position many times, and it's no fun. Injuries, illness and unexpected events happen. They are just part of life. When it comes to fitness, nutrition and wellness plans, it's important to remember that it's not "all or nothing". Flexibility and patience are key factors to success over the long run.

Be Gentle With Yourself

When we are sick or injured, our bodies need down-time to recover and heal, especially in the acute stages. An inability to exercise doesn't mean your entire "master wellness plan" needs to be thrown out the window. In fact, it's probably more important than ever to zone in on your nutrition and ensure you are eating a nourishing array of foods that will help your body heal. Don't allow your disappointment and frustration to lead you to the freezer for a late night ice cream binge. Seek out other ways to boost both your body and your injured ego. Look for gentle wellness behaviours that you can engage in while you recover.

- Get a massage.
- Try gentle stretching if it is possible.
- Read a book about nutrition.
- Read healthy recipe books or blogs and get inspired by the drool-worthy photos.
- Meditate on topics that might be relevant like patience and self-compassion.
- Stay hydrated.
- Stay committed to any physiotherapy or rehabilitation exercises you may have been prescribed. (Does anyone else struggle with this one?!)
- Go for a gentle stroll if you can.

Be Flexible

If you are injured, you still might be able to engage in a gentler form of movement. (Always consult with your health care provider first.) I was in a minor car accident a few years ago and suffered a concussion and neck injury. Running and lifting weights were completely out of the question for many months. I was extremely frustrated, discouraged and depressed. Although I missed my regular fitness routine, I still found small ways to be active (all cleared by my physiotherapist). I was still able to walk. Some days, all I could muster was a trip to the end of my driveway. Even this small amount of movement at least got my muscles and joints moving and lifted my spirits.

I also suffered a debilitating case of tennis elbow that lingered for close to a year. During this time, I simply focused on activities that involved my lower body. I was able to run and cycle pain free. Eventually, I was even able to work in certain weighted upper body moves that didn't irritate my injury.

Moving forward with your goals at a slower pace is a much better option than putting on the brakes and allowing yourself to slide back downhill! Although following that twelve week bikini body program to a tee is no longer on the table, a flexible mindset will allow you to seek alternatives so you can remain active. Maybe you were a runner in your youth, but your bad knee no longer allows you to pound the pavement. Why not think outside the box so you can keep moving? Maybe swimming or water aerobics would be gentler on your joints.

Have a Plan B

I think back-up plans are incredibly useful in many areas of life, but particularly when it comes to keeping your health and wellness goals on track. Having a reliable *Plan B* that you can turn to when things don't go your way is always a better option than throwing in the towel.

Let's say you and your girlfriend were planning to meet up after work for a walk. The sidewalks are slick from an unexpected episode of freezing rain in the afternoon, so you cancel your plans in the interest of safety. Certainly, this is a legitimate excuse to take a pass on walking, but it doesn't mean you can't reach for another option. The two of you could meet at a local gym and share a fitness class together. You could also opt to just head home and tune in to an online HIIT training session. There are literally a zillion at-home workouts available online. Bookmark your favorites and pull them out when the need arises.

Let's say you planned a very healthy meal for this evening's dinner, but your last meeting of the day ran very late. You arrive home frazzled and famished. The meal you had arranged for tonight's menu is going to take at least forty-five minutes to pull together. In times like these, it's great to have healthy Plan B options on hand that can be ready to serve in minutes. I keep my freezer stocked with hearty soups and stews that can be quickly defrosted and on the table in no time. Having a few pre-made salads in the refrigerator can also be saviours in a pinch. (I discuss meal planning and prepping in greater detail in chapter 6.) An inventory of Plan B meals will save you from having to call for pizza delivery!

Having a variety of Plan B's in your back pocket allows you to be flexible. They serve as safeguards against unexpected circumstances.

Have Portable Options

Do you find it difficult to stick to your health plans when you leave the comfort and security of your regular schedule? Travelling for work or play can often throw us off track. Routines are broken, and access to our regular food and activities can be restricted.

I'm always sure to pack my health goals in my suitcase when I leave home (yes, even on vacation). I'm not trying to be a downer. Because eating well and exercising make me feel good, I never want to leave them behind! It doesn't mean that I don't indulge in treats when on vacation, it just means that I don't go hog wild. I take a balanced approach; indulging in a few special treats while still main-taining an overall mindset of healthy eating. I seek out healthy choices on menus, and I pack nutritious snacks to tide me over during times where options are limited.

Most vacations our family takes include activities, because we are all naturally an active bunch. (My two boys don't sit still for long.) That being said, I never forget to pack my running shoes. I still get up early to enjoy a morning walk, run or small workout routine (no equipment required). It allows me to start the day feeling fresh and energized and ready for adventure. I've also had the luxury of going on some of the most beautiful runs of my life on vacation. Running the meandering back roads of the French countryside, listening to the birds and soaking in the pastoral views is a memory I hold close to my heart.

I encourage you carry on with your healthy lifestyle choices, even when travelling. Take a balanced approach that will allow you to stick to your goals while still enjoying fun foods and activities.

Consistency is Key

In the grand scheme of things, consistency is key when it comes to adopting healthy lifestyle habits. We are all going to experience ups and downs. I picture my own graph of healthy living as a rolling wave of highs and lows. During my low times, I'm conscious not to let the bottom fall out. *It's not all or nothing.* Having a crappy day doesn't have to spiral into a crappy week or a crappy month. Regroup, rethink and keep moving forward!

Elevating Actions and Inspiration

- Avoid the trap of all-or-nothing thinking when it comes to your health, fitness and nutrition goals. If you find yourself in an unfortunate situation that is preventing you from following through on certain healthy actions, don't give up on everything. Any small step towards better health is a good choice.

- During times of illness or injury, carry on as best you can with other healthy habits. If an injury has you laid up or you are under the weather, make sure you are still eating a nutritious diet. If you aren't feeling up for a run, but can swing something gentler like stretching, pull out that yoga mat. Look for small, gentle ways to keep moving forward with your goals.

- Keep an open mind and choose to be flexible and creative if you are no longer able to perform certain favorite activities. Focus on methods of exercise that don't involve your injured body part! Get creative and try something new that doesn't aggravate your aches and pains.

- Have a Plan B in the back of your mind that you can reach for when things don't go as planned. It's useful to have a list of indoor fitness activities you can turn to if you are someone who frequently exercises outdoors. Don't let the weather serve as an excuse to miss a workout!

- Having an inventory of Plan B meals on hand is a great way to prevent last minute calls for unhealthy take out. When you are tired, running late or just feeling lazy, a stash of premade health food will keep you on track with your nutrition goals.

- Carry your health goals and aspirations with you wherever you go! Before heading on vacation or a work-related trip, put a little thought into how you can maintain your healthy habits while traveling. Plan ahead for fitness activities, which could include walking, running, using a hotel fitness facility or doing a simple exercise routine that doesn't require equipment. Pack healthy snacks and seek out healthy menu options.

- Keep in mind that consistency is key. Small setbacks don't need to completely sidetrack your efforts. A flexible, open-minded and committed approach to your health is the key to success!

6

INSPIRE YOURSELF IN
THE KITCHEN

When it comes to healthy eating, I have found the key to staying on track is to keep things simple and easy, but also fun and inspiring. Life is busy for all of us, and I've learned that you don't need to be a professional chef, or have a passion for cooking to eat a diet of healthy, delicious and uplifting foods.

Cooking is really not one of my hobbies. I would much rather spend time working on my creative pursuits or getting outside and being active. To be truthful, if given the choice, I would enjoy a day of cleaning and organizing my house more than time at the cooktop. Despite this, I do have a passion for eating a healthy diet that feels nourishing to both my body and my soul.

Maybe you are a master of the kitchen! If this is the case, go ahead and use this to your advantage. Seek out ways to combine your passion for food preparation with your interest in wellness and nutrition.

I believe that as human beings, we instinctively want to eat nutritious foods. When our bodies are in a healthy state they crave foods that promote wellbeing and vitality. My body is certainly loud and clear when I've opted for a choice that it doesn't agree with. I have two "weak spots" my body chooses to communicate through when it is feeling a bit perturbed with my food choices. My digestive system is super sensitive. An overindulgence in anything irritating to my system is going to hit me straight in the gut. I also have a history of terrible throat infections, and my tonsils are always keen to make me aware when I'm getting run-down.

Unfortunately, we humans are also our own worst enemies! As a society, we have created such an overwhelming, abundant and tempting selection of absolute crap food that we are bombarded with at every turn. It can definitely be tough to navigate through the minefield of junk food, especially when we are feeling tired, stressed and pressed for time. Fast food drive-throughs, convenient processed foods, greasy cafeteria options, eye-pleasing candy displays...there is no escaping these seductive temptations.

With a bit of planning, effort and the right mindset, I believe all of us have the ability stay committed to a nutritious diet by simply making it a part of our lifestyle. It's not about going on a diet, but rather adopting a healthy way of eating that is sustainable, satisfying, joyful and nourishing. It's about finding a system that works for *your* lifestyle, personality and preferences. It's about dreaming up and adopting a set strategies that will set *you* up for success! You need to feel a true sense of enthusiasm for adopting a healthy lifestyle, and finding ways to motivate and inspire yourself can really be a game changer in sticking with things for the long haul.

What works for one person might not work for the next. Ask yourself what roadblocks you personally encounter when attempting to eat in a healthier manner, and from there try to dream up some creative, yet practical solutions. I think the key to setting yourself up for success is creating an environment that inspires you to make healthy choices, but that also makes it feel effortless!

I pulled together a list of my own challenges to share with you. You might identify and connect with me on some, all, or none of these!

- Feeling uninspired when I open my fridge and cupboards.
- Finding something quick and satisfying to eat when I'm famished.
- Trying to come up with healthy meal ideas that will please all (or at least most) members of my family.
- Dealing with unexpected situations where I don't have the time or energy to prepare the meal I had planned.

It's a worthwhile exercise to analyze your own situation and create a personalized list. This will present you with a starting point to brainstorm creative solutions for your issues. Here's what I came up with:

Create an Enticing Display

Let's get really honest with ourselves here. What is the state of your refrigerator? When you open the door, are you inspired and uplifted by the overflowing bounty of crisp produce staring you in the face? Are healthy snacks at your fingertips, easy to grab and go? Are you stocked up with a fresh array of enticing ingredients, making it a breeze to whip up a quick and nutritious meal? Is the scene perhaps a little less inspiring than this aspirational image? I will admit, my fridge was in a pretty nasty state a couple of weeks ago. It had reached the point where it was jam packed, but it felt like we had no food in the house. I'm guessing this might sound familiar to some of you!

In my book *Elevate Your Personal Style,* I have a chapter titled "Merchandise Your Products". I suggest that if you want to motivate yourself to dress well each day, it helps if you display your clothing and accessories in a pleasing and inspiring manner. Essentially, I recommend turning your wardrobe into your own personal chic boutique! With your pretty scarves on display, and your clothing neatly hung and organized, you will be more likely to reach for a creative and uplifting outfit!

Why not take the same approach when it comes to your refrigerator? Why not merchandise your healthy foods so they are presented in an enticing and convenient manner, just like an attractive deli display or market stand? This approach really works wonders in my household, and I always feel more productive and in a healthy mindset when I'm following my own advice. Not only am I better able to come up with healthy meal ideas, but my family is more likely to reach for a nutritious snack if healthy options are in plain view and require no effort to grab. (I'll be honest, no one in my house is going to take the initiative to pull a knife from the drawer and cut up a watermelon. If, however, it is sliced and on display, it's always the first thing to go!)

I finally rolled up my sleeves and did a complete deep clean and overhaul of my fridge. I felt so much lighter and so much more enthusiastic about spending time in the kitchen. When you open the door and your food is neatly and attractively arranged, you have a clear view of what you have on hand! There is no need to dig through produce drawers, or tentatively open that plastic container hiding behind the pickles. It just plain feels good to have a clean, organized fridge stocked with fresh food!

What if your pantry looked like the shelves of your favorite health food store? I picked up some inexpensive glass jars, and instead of storing my dry goods (rice, lentils, oatmeal) in the original packaging, I have everything displayed in an antique cupboard. Having those brightly colored lentils in plain view inspires me to actually incorporate them into my cooking on a regular basis! In addition, it is just more enjoyable to scoop something out of a solid jar instead of fiddling with a bag. Taking an afternoon to clean out and organize your cupboards really can be an invigorating project that can kickstart you on a path to better eating and more inspired cooking. (I *did* mention I actually *enjoy* cleaning and organizing!)

Adopt a Salad Bar Approach

Finding yourself in a state of being famished usually doesn't end well…unless you are prepared! Instead of relying on that old familiar standby for a quick hit of food, (which for me tends to be a giant bowl of cereal) what if you had much healthier snack and meal options all pre-prepped and conveniently on hand? What if you opened your fridge to find your very own *salad bar* inside, with all the ingredients ready and waiting for you to concoct a quick and healthy plate of food?

Instead of reaching for that cereal box, you could treat yourself to a colorful plate of pre-cut veggies and hummus. You could take two minutes and top a bowl of greens and veggies (already washed and cut) with a satisfying serving of your protein of choice, a sprinkling of seeds and nuts and some tasty dressing. Let's face it, it feels a lot easier to dump a pile of flakes in a bowl than it does to take the time to peel and chop a carrot. Having those carrots sticks (and peppers slices, broccoli florets, celery sticks and cucumber slices) already prepped makes choosing the healthier option a lot easier.

I like to set aside a bit of time each week to assemble my salad bar and create an assortment of ready-to-go snack and quick meal options. There is nothing complicated about this. You could designate an hour on a Sunday afternoon

Elevate Your Health

to this task, or you could commit to doing a bit of chopping before you put the groceries away. Here is a sample of prepped food I like to keep on hand. (I eat a plant-based diet, so my list could be amended to include something like pre-cooked shredded chicken to suit your needs.)

- An assortment of chopped veggies along with containers of hummus on hand
- Washed and cut up fruit (melon, berries, pineapple, grapes)
- Washed apples on display (so easy, yet my children will only eat them if they can actually see them)
- Cooked quinoa
- Cooked lentils
- Cooked wild rice
- Drained and rinsed black beans and chickpeas (Yes, the task of opening a can feels like a lot of effort at times, so having this done with the beans ready for eating is helpful.)
- Washed and cut up greens for salads (kale, spinach, mixed lettuces)
- Shredded carrots and cabbage
- Roasted nuts and pumpkin seeds (A few minutes under the broiler really brings out their flavour.)
- A jar or two of my favorite homemade salad dressings

My salad bar has saved me more times than I can count. I can't imagine running my kitchen without it!

:: 53 ::

Please Yourself and Your Family

Cooking for a family can be challenging, especially when people have different likes and tastes. As a mother myself, I can now appreciate what I put my own mother through as a child. I was a very picky eater!

When it comes to children, I know many people are of the mindset that we should not cater to their likes and dislikes. They should eat what is put in front of them. I think because I disliked a lot of foods as a child, I'm a bit more sensitive and empathetic to those who genuinely don't like certain foods. Should we be forced to eat something that tastes or feels unpleasant to us? I think trying new foods is important, but presenting my family with healthy foods they truly love and enjoy on a regular basis is what feels right for me.

How do I create meals to please everyone around the table? I certainly don't every day, but I try my best to make everyone reasonably happy. I pull out the salad bar approach regularly! For instance, let's say I planned a Mediterranean falafel bowl for dinner. This would include a salad of cucumbers, tomatoes, greens and olives. I would serve a side of brown rice and roasted chickpeas along with the falafel. Toppings would include a vinaigrette dressing, hummus, chopped parsley and cilantro and crumbled feta. (My children eat dairy now and then even though my husband and I don't.) If it were just my husband and me, I'd mix up the salad, throw on the toppings and dinner would be served. Instead, I set the whole thing up as a salad bar on the counter. The kids can therefore create their own plates. One child hates tomatoes, the other doesn't like cilantro. Both my husband and I take a pass on the feta. Everyone gets to assemble a meal that suits their taste and include or omit items as they please. I find that the kids are more likely to eat what's on their plates, because they were involved in the decision making. Any leftovers are just added to my selection of pre-cut and prepared fridge inventory, to be used for the next day's lunch or a snack.

Something else I really enjoy getting creative with is seeking out recipes for healthier versions of more traditional meals. Going vegan has actually been a fun and challenging project that has allowed me to convert old-standby meals into something more nutritious. We all love my version of plant-based macaroni and cheese. It is made with a base of carrots, cashews, almond milk and nutritional yeast. It's creamy and tasty and much healthier than the old-style recipe loaded with butter and greasy cheese. I've also got a great kale Caesar salad recipe that I believe rivals the original!

Make a list of some of your family's favorite meals and have fun researching alternative recipes that use healthier ingredients. It really is possible to create a family menu that both appeals to everyone's taste and health goals.

Have a Plan A and a Plan B

I touched on the concept of having a *Plan B* in the previous chapter. This of course assumes that you have a

Plan A in the first place! When it comes to healthy eating, Plan A represents your best intentions and your ideal blueprint for your week of eating. This is basically your meal plan!

Meal planning is such a wonderful tool to keep us on track with our healthy eating. Grocery shopping with that meal plan in hand ensures that you have all the ingredients at your fingertips when you need them. Having a plan really helps life run more smoothly, especially during particularly busy times of the year. I'm always looking for ways to reduce stress in my life, and being proactive with meal planning is usually top on my list of priorities.

I might argue, however, that Plan B is just as, if not more important than Plan A in keeping you on track. Plan B comes in handy when you need it the most and during your weakest moments. It keeps you from derailing all your grand plans and allows you to stay on course with your goals, even when the unexpected happens. It will save you a hundred times from just reaching for the take-out menu.

As I mentioned in chapter 5, having a small inventory of healthy freezer meals is a great Plan B that you can rely on time and time again. Another Plan B in my house is that salad bar system I use. On nights where defrosting a meal even feels like too much effort, digging out my salad bar can save the day. Having a "design your own plate" style of meal is actually a fun option that allows everyone to dig into what they are craving. It's also a great way to use up leftovers. Plan B might mean keeping a stash of nuts and health bars in the car to snack on when you are tied up running errands longer than expected. Anything you can do to set yourself up to stay on track deserves a Plan B title!

Elevating Actions and Inspiration

- Set yourself up for success with your nutrition goals. Take some time to identify the roadblocks or challenges you face when it comes to staying on track with healthy eating. Seek out fun and creative ways to inspire yourself to eat well. Keep things simple and easy for the best results.

- Set some time aside to clean out your refrigerator and pantry. Have fun organizing and displaying your food in an attractive manner. Not only will you have a clearer view of what's in stock, but you will be more inspired to eat those nutritious goodies.

- Turn your fridge into your personal salad bar, complete with all your favorite toppings. This can become your convenience food instead of a box of crackers.

- If you are in charge of preparing meals for others, look for solutions that will please everyone. Allowing others to assemble their own plates is a great strategy in keeping everyone happy.

- Have fun researching healthier alternatives to traditional family favorites. The revised versions are often just as tasty as the originals (often better!)
- Plan your meals and grocery shop accordingly. Knowing ahead of time what is on the menu and having all the ingredients on hand is usually half the battle
- Have a Plan B in place for when the unexpected occurs. Keep a little stash of meals tucked away in your freezer. Ensure your fridge is always stocked with the bare essentials to whip up Buddha bowl style meal. If you are tied up in traffic, running late at work, or just plain exhausted, Plan B options can be lifesavers.

7

TREAD LIGHTLY WITH TREATS

I wasn't a particularly rebellious teenager. Most people who knew me back in the day would have likely classified me as a bit of a "goody-two-shoes". (Honestly, things haven't changed that much in thirty years.) I didn't smoke or drink in high school. I guess I expressed my defiance through food, and more specifically, sugar, fat and salt (my drugs of choice). Growing up with a mother trained in nutrition, I had to go out of my way to feed my addictions!

I'm about to reveal a couple of secrets that are likely going to hurt my dear mother's heart. (Sorry Mom…kids can be jerks!) She put her heart and soul into providing our family with healthy meals. She packed me the most beautiful, thoughtful, nutritious lunches for twelve straight years. As a mother myself now, I realize that this was one of the ways she expressed her love for me. This makes my confession here even more painful and heart-wrenching to admit.

Starting in grade nine, every single one of those lunches ended up in the trash (or more accurately, the bottom of my locker...and then the trash, after complaints of a foul stench were lodged against me). I just did the math, (accountant here) and that adds up to about eight hundred lunches. Most days I skipped my way down to the cafeteria to order a steaming plate of poutine (a Canadian speciality of French fries topped with gravy and cheese curds). Because my mom was a teacher at the school and often on lunch duty, I had to strategically place the plate in front of a friend, so she didn't discover my dirty little secret.

When my best friend and I were looking for trouble, we usually ended up in the kitchen. In our grade eleven year we became obsessed with brown sugar fudge. We were whipping up batches of fudge so often, that my mother eventually stepped in and banned us from making it! As with anything forbidden, the naughtiness factor made us crave it all the more. We mischievously looked for any opportunity to throw together a batch in secret. I remember heavily dousing the kitchen in Windex to try to mask the evidence and odor of our deceitful acts! We beat the fudge in my bedroom, where we then proceeded to eat the entire sticky mess, straight from the pot!

I'm not proud of these admissions, but it goes to show just how addictive junk food is! I mentioned in the previous chapter that I believe our bodies crave nutritious foods when we are in a balanced state of health. On the other hand, when we allow ourselves to get off kilter, and indulge in treat foods too often, it seems the opposite is true. I realize there is lots of science around all this, but to simplify it, I just have to look to my own experience. The more junk I eat, the more junk I crave. The healthier I eat, the more healthy foods I crave.

With all that being said, I do believe that food is one of the greatest joys in life. We all have favorite treats that we look forward to eating, and I personally don't see any harm in indulging in them occasionally if my overall diet is nutritious. The key, however, is to keep things in check, and not take things to the extreme. Depriving yourself of all your favorite treats and junk food is one definition of extreme. Binging on them regularly with wild abandon also falls into the extreme category. Ideally, you find a way to live in a happy state of balance, where you nourish your body daily with a variety and fresh and healthy foods, and allow yourself on occasion to dip into your guilty pleasures (without guilt).

We're all human! It's so easy to fall prey to temptation in weak moments and lose sight of our wellness goals. It's certainly not that one moment of weakness is going to throw our health into chaos. It's more about the sum of all our small daily choices, and how much their effects accumulate over time.

Over the years, I've been able to identify my own areas of weakness, and I've developed a set of personal strategies that allow me to tread lightly on treats without feeling deprived. I'm certainly not perfect in this department, but I feel that I strike a happy balance. My goal is to eat in a manner that promotes wellness, vitality, longevity *and* enjoyment. Here are a few tips that help set me up for success!

Adopt a Just-In-Time Inventory System

I apologize for pulling out the accounting terminology, but I couldn't resist. "Just-in-time" perfectly describes my approach to stocking my shelves with treat foods. You can probably guess that a business using a just-in-time inventory management system only receives goods into its warehouse when they are needed for production or sale. Why not take the same approach with your kitchen cupboards? It's a lot easier to make healthy choices when junk food isn't on the premises.

I am a planner (no surprise). I grew up as a proud member of the Girl Guides of Canada, and I took their motto, "Be Prepared" very seriously. I don't usually promote procrastination, however I'm going to encourage you to throw this concept out the window when it comes to food shopping for special events, occasions and holidays.

Let's use Halloween as an example. Stocking up early means the treats are lying around your house, calling your name for weeks or days before the big day. It's easy to convince yourself that "one little treat" is no big deal every time you pass by the stash. Before long, you've eaten three quarters of a bag of Rockets and Halloween is still four days away!

I don't think there is a grave threat that the stores are going to run out of treats before the 31st. Why not pick them up at the very last moment, and save yourself from the torment of having treats easily accessible for the period leading up to Halloween night?

You can adopt the just-in-time mindset for ordinary, everyday occasions as well. If you are planning a family movie night on Friday and a few treats are in order, pick them up that evening on the way home from work, instead of including them in the weekly grocery order.

Ignore the Economics

As an accountant, I'm fully aware that buying in bulk is a money-saving strategy that helps decrease the cost-per-unit price. In fact, a few years ago I ran a small bulk buying group with some friends from my community. We used to buy pallets worth of dry goods at wholesale prices and divvy them up between us. We bought everything from flour, to oatmeal, quinoa, lentils, nuts, seeds, dried fruit and olive oil! We saved a ton of money, and kept our pantry shelves stocked with a wide variety of high quality, healthy ingredients.

Once again, however, I'm going to go against my instincts and recommend something I wouldn't normally consider under normal circumstances. While I believe we should attempt to stretch every dollar in our grocery budget, I think we should adopt the opposite approach when it comes to junk food! Yes, it's cheaper to take advantage of the two-for-one deal on the soda pop. Yes, the cost per gram is more attractive on the family sized bag of chips. Fight that inner accountant inside you (we all have one) and choose to buy *just enough*. Buy just enough ice cream to complement the birthday cake with none left over. Buy just enough chips for each member of the family to enjoy a reasonable serving on movie night.

Shopping with a *just enough* mindset in the treat section really goes hand in hand with the just-in-time system. Together, they create a winning combination to keep junky foods out of reach (and therefore out of your mouth) most days!

Don't be Shy to be a Little Selfish

It might sound mean spirited to suggest that you offer treats you don't even like to others, but we all have different tastes! Your least favorite candy bar might be someone else's treasure! I used to have a weakness for Tootsie Rolls because they were one of my most-loved penny candies growing up. Each Halloween, I found myself reaching for this nostalgic favorite when selecting candy to hand out to our community. Their mere presence was too hard to pass up, and I soon found myself indulging in them to excess. One year I just decided to stop buying them! Why put myself through the misery? I'm not a fan of chocolate bars and sour candies, so I reach for those instead these days. Since I don't even like them, the idea of treating myself to one of them isn't even appealing!

Getting selfish during holidays where treats are abundant isn't about being a party pooper. I don't think anyone in my house ever feels shortchanged by Santa or the Easter Bunny (and with our one thousand foot driveway, we often don't even have trick-or-treaters ringing the doorbell). Again, it's really about adopting an approach that sets *you* up for success. By identifying your weak spots, you can approach special events with a more mindful and planned approach.

It's Not All-or-Nothing

I already touched on all-or-nothing thinking in chapter 5, but it's worth revisiting in the context of treats. Have you ever caught yourself during a binge and thought, "It's too late now! I might as well finish off the entire tin of cookies since I've eaten half a dozen already." I'm pretty sure I may have adopted this mindset with those Tootsie Rolls!

You can't change the past, (the cookies you've already consumed) but you can change how you behave in the present moment. You make the rules. At any given moment, you can adjust your sails and change your course. You don't have to get lost and drown in that bag of chips my friend! You have the ability and the choice to stop, regroup and reconnect with the vision of elevated health you envisaged in chapter 1.

Create Personalized Strategies

This is a good time to pull out the wellness journal and reconnect with your "why's" and all the inspiring and motivational content you created for yourself. It's also a worthwhile exercise to give some thought to your own frustrations surrounding food. Where and when do you feel most vulnerable to fall off the wagon? What occasions, situations and emotions bring about cravings for large doses of junk food? What temptations are the hardest for you to resist?

If you are someone who reaches for comfort food when you are feeling stressed or down, I encourage you to seek out more elevating approaches to healing your heart. In my book, *Elevate the Everyday,* I included a chapter called "Self Soothe in an Uplifting Manner". I created a list of healthy ideas we can all reach for when we need a little pick me up (instead of that second slice of chocolate cake).

Hopefully the ideas I've provided here will help get you started on creating your own list of personal strategies to enjoy those special treats using a balanced, healthy and reasonable approach.

Elevating Actions and Inspiration

- Keep temptations at bay by adopting a just-in-time inventory mindset around treat foods. It's more likely you will make unhealthy food choices if junk food is easily accessible and on hand at your weakest moments. Buy any treats you need for a special event or planned occasion at the very last minute. Otherwise, keep the stock levels at zero!

- Resist the urge to save your pennies and buy in bulk when it comes to junk food. Buy *just enough* to fill your need. Don't allow for any leftovers!

- Who says you always have to treat others to *your* personal favorites? Avoid bringing personal junk food favorites into the home if possible.

- If you find yourself heading down the road to "Bingeville", slam on the brakes and remind yourself it's never all or nothing. You get to set the rules and have the power to stop at the halfway mark if you want to.

- Take some time to identify your own areas of weakness. Use inspiration from this book as a starting point to create your own list of strategies to keep you on track with healthy food choices.

8

THINK ACTIVE, NOT ATHLETIC

Are you someone who played sports all your life? Maybe you were a gymnast, a basketball player or a competitive swimmer (or all of the above). Do you consider yourself a natural athlete? Maybe you find yourself on the other end of the spectrum. You were always the kid with her nose in a book. You dreaded gym class, and shied away from all sports and active pursuits. "I'm so clumsy! I hate exercise. I don't have an athletic bone in my body. I don't like sweating and gasping for air!" Do any of these statements sound familiar?

Most of us probably fall somewhere in the middle. I was definitely a bookworm as a child, but I was also very active and outdoorsy. I enjoyed being out in nature and spent my days riding my bike, skipping, climbing trees and exploring the woods and hills behind our home. I played a few team sports in junior high and high school. I wasn't particularly talented at them, but I enjoyed the comradery that went along with being a member of a team. I would classify myself as your average, everyday kid.

As a mother, I can certainly acknowledge that organized sport offers a wide array of positive outcomes; physical, mental and social. One of my sons plays competitive soccer. His speed, agility, strength and cardiovascular fitness are certainly impressive. I notice the positive impact the team environment has on his self-esteem and confidence. Certainly, there are many life lessons to be learned through competitive sport. That being said, it's really important to embrace the concept of physical activity, outside the realm of competition.

As childhood obesity rates continue to rise, I wonder where we are missing the mark. Would a greater focus on being *active* versus *athletic* help the situation? Both of my boys played hockey for a few years, and I always cringed when the sponsoring donut shop in town (I'm not naming names, but if you are Canadian, you know exactly who I'm referring to) offered free hot chocolate if you showed up at their restaurant wearing your jersey. After a healthy hour of physical activity, here they are encouraging our children to guzzle back more calories than they just expended. (Please don't get me started on sports drinks.)

Somehow I think society as a whole is giving and receiving the wrong message. Many kids leave their one-hour sports sessions, only to go home and plop on the couch with a video game console (said sports drink in hand). I'd love to see society put more money and focus on teaching our kids how to embrace *self-directed physical activity.* They would then have a solid base to carry forward to adulthood.

Interestingly, my children absolutely thrived during the pandemic, despite the fact all their formal sporting activities were cancelled. They spent their days riding their mountain bikes and building trails. (Manual labour is hard work!)

Stop Keeping Score

I've noticed that there are mental traps to fall into no matter where you sit on the spectrum of physical talents and tendencies. I think one of the most important keys in both embracing and maintaining an active lifestyle is to identify more with the word *active* versus *athletic*. At the end of the day, you can be one of the most talented athletes on earth, but if you aren't actually out there moving your body, it's not going to do you a stitch of good in the health department. I can think of a number of people who were star athletes in their youth, only to let it all slide during mid-life. I've noticed that many adults still associate activity with team or organized sport (a carryforward from childhood no doubt). The heavy focus on competitive sports growing up didn't allow for much time or attention to develop active hobbies and interests off the field, rink or court.

I often hear adults lament that they only feel inspired to engage in team sports, or participate in activities in the company of others. (My husband, a former high-performing athlete, has brought up this point many, many times!) This attitude can set you up for potential roadblocks.

Adults lead busy lives, so it can be difficult to consistently and reliably fit these types of activities into your day. I'm not at all saying that you shouldn't participate in group activities! I'm a huge advocate of doing what you love. If you love basketball, then find a pickup league and play! Do what makes you happy and what you will be most motivated to participate in.

It is also a good idea, however, to balance things out by finding activities where you don't need to rely on others. Taking a mixed bag approach will help you stay on track with fitness goals, because you offer yourself more options, and therefore fewer excuses. Cycling, running, walking, hiking, weightlifting, and swimming can all be rewarding solo activities that offer the benefit of flexibility. If your indoor soccer league is cancelled, or you are running late at work and miss bootcamp, it is nice to have a repertoire of other activities to choose from.

While I am a big fan of workout buddies (I had a running partner for many years), the only person you can count on 100% of the time to show up is yourself! Don't restrict your own efforts by adopting the mindset that you can only exercise if someone is watching or keeping score. Opening your mind will open doors and opportunities!

Don't Sell Yourself Short

I'm going to repeat what I just said above – opening your mind will open doors and opportunities. If you are one of those people who has always avoided exercise because you feel clumsy, awkward, or inadequate, this statement could also be helpful to you. Shifting your mindset to an active versus athletic approach will help you realize that you don't have to be "good" at an activity to experience enjoyment and health benefits from it.

While I certainly admire the natural gifts and hard work put in by talented athletes, I'm more impressed by the everyday heroes out there. It's the regular people who embrace an active mindset throughout their lives that really fascinate and motivate me. I love drawing inspiration from people who aren't necessarily athletically gifted, (sorry Dad, but this is you) but who have maintained an active lifestyle straight through into their golden years. I admire those individuals who keep moving forward, despite the obstacles in their path. This includes people like my cousin, who continued to stay active with weights and yoga during his cancer treatments. My former Girl Guide leader intrigues me. She is still going strong at the age of ninety something, despite a heart valve replacement decades ago. (Not a day went by growing up that I didn't see her out for her walk.) Focusing on the act, versus the score or competition, allows all these individuals to embrace an active, healthy mindset.

It doesn't matter if you are running at the back of the pack. It doesn't matter if you are the most uncoordinated person in dance class (definitely me in tap dancing). It doesn't matter if you find yourself reaching for the tiny dumbbells, while the beast of a woman next to you is grabbing the heaviest ones on site! What matters is that you are being active, moving your body and experiencing the endless benefits of exercise as a result. Taking action can only keep you moving in the right direction towards better health.

Turn Hate Into Love

Over the years, I have heard many people claim how much they hate exercise, and running in particular. I felt the same way about running, before I became an avid runner myself. I'll never forget the dreaded annual "Endurance Run" in gym class. Every year we were required to participate in the "Canada Fitness Awards" program through the school system. This involved performing a series of fitness tests, which was always capped off with being forced to run at least a hundred laps around the gym. (It was probably less than that, but you get the point.) I hated every single minute of it. It's hard to believe ten years later I found myself running a marathon.

If you are a self-professed "exercise-hater", I encourage you to dig a little deeper into the underlying thoughts and feelings around your attitude. I thought I hated running, but once I dipped my toe into it, I realized I actually enjoyed it. I realized what I hated about running was the terrible feeling of gasping for air that any newbie to the sport is going to experience. I never really gave myself a chance to like it, because I always quit as soon as things got a little uncomfortable. When I finally gave it the fair chance it deserved, I realized that those "out of breath" sensations pass in time, and they are replaced with feelings of exhilaration, strength and energy.

I've never been a big fan of the "no pain, no gain" expression, but there is a bit of truth to it. My advice is to start any new activity gently, and give yourself time to warm up to it. You might be pleasantly surprised like I was.

Make New Friends

Changing your relationship with exercise is another approach that can be helpful in shifting your mindset. If you are someone who claims to hate exercise, try reframing your self-talk around physical activity. Adopting a mindset of gratitude can be very uplifting! Replace "I *have* to work out" with "I *get* to work out". Yay! You get to participate in something that will leave you feeling strong, invigorated and energized. It's a much more pleasant and elevating mindset than begrudgingly taking part in what you view as just another dreaded chore.

I actually view my running as a *friend*. It's been a constant and faithful companion of mine for over twenty years. It's always there when I need it; reliable and quietly non-judgemental. It has seen me through some of the darkest periods of my life. It dragged me out of bed and got me moving on days when I didn't see the point. It never leaves my side. It has accompanied me through the familiar streets of my own neighbourhood, as well as on meandering jaunts through picturesque foreign villages. It has lifted my spirits, and given me confidence and strength (from the inside out). It has listened to my anger and allowed me to vent unapologetically. It is patient with me when I'm feeling a little tired and sore, always willing to slow the pace if necessary. It knows when I need a push, and challenges me to reach new heights. Running (and exercise in general) is a true friend, that elevates my life on so many levels.

Wouldn't you too like to have such a faithful companion in your life? It almost sounds too good to be true, but it is something that is available to each and every one of us. Imaginary friends of this sort are free and accessible to all. Physical activity is a generous friend that only gives, and never takes. I encourage you to get out there and add a few new friendships to your inner circle!

Elevating Actions and Inspiration

- By identifying with the word *active* versus athletic, we are more likely to keep an open mind when it comes to participating in physical fitness activities.
- If you are someone who has always relied on team or competitive environments to motivate you to participate, shifting your focus to *activity* can allow for more flexibility in your life. With more options at your fingertips, you are more likely to be consistent with your efforts. You will not need to rely solely on the presence of others for motivation.

- Realize that you don't have to excel at an activity or sport in order to reap benefits from it. The health benefits associated with physical activity stem from participation! Don't let your insecurities or pre-conceived notions about your talents hold you back from enjoying an active lifestyle.

- Give your workouts a fair shot! Many people quit before they give the benefits of an activity a chance to kick in. Open your mind to the fact that those activities you claim to hate might in fact offer powerful and elevating benefits. It's a lot easier to turn that hate into love (or even like) than you think!

- View exercise as a friend. Approach it with a mind-set of gratitude and be thankful that you have a body that is able to participate in it. Holding a grudge against it is surely going to make the experience unpleasant.

9

DISCOVER WHAT MAKES YOU TICK

What lights you up inside? What gets your fire burning? Doing a bit of self-discovery to identify what inspires you can be a game changer. By having a better understanding of what makes you tick, you can develop strategies to keep yourself motivated and moving forward with your health goals.

When it comes to motivating myself, I like to draw on a number of different approaches. If you are like me, you might need to mix things up depending on your mood or the situation. We all react differently to situations, so the key is to find out what works for *you*. Here are a few tactics I have found to be helpful over the years with keeping myself on track with my goals. Hopefully, some of these will resonate with you!

Reward Yourself

Who doesn't like winning prizes? While we can't do much about our chances on that lottery ticket, we can treat ourselves regularly to rewards for our efforts. In my book, *Elevate the Everyday,* I discuss how I use a dreamy/ practical approach when compiling my to do list for the day. My list includes practical tasks, interspersed with dreamy and enjoyable activities. I regularly reward myself with a dreamy task, once I complete one of my practical tasks. For instance, after I update the household finances and pay the bills, I reward myself with a moment of downtime to sip my tea and scroll through pretty pictures on Pinterest.

The same approach can be used if you are someone who needs a little nudge to get out of bed or off the couch to get moving. What if you told yourself that after that workout, you will treat yourself to a moment of delicious-ness? What constitutes a reward will look different to everyone. For you it might be a hot cup of coffee and some guilt-free time to check in on your favorite blogs. For someone else, it might mean enjoying a few extra soothing minutes in a hot shower. Although I prefer to stay away from "treat foods" as rewards, I do view my healthy foods as something to look forward too. For instance, I love my breakfast of oatmeal and blueberries so much, I consider it my post-run reward. I prefer to run on an empty stomach, so coming home to my yummy breakfast and morning tea is a treat that I savour.

Grab your journal and dream up a list of petite treats and rewards that you can indulge in after a job well done. Here are a few ideas to get your started:

- Take a long hot shower
- Read a chapter of the book on your nightstand
- Give yourself a mini-manicure and fresh coat of polish
- Take a soothing bath and apply a face mask
- Take a nap
- Scroll through inspiring Pinterest boards
- Read your favorite blogs
- Arrange a bouquet of wildflowers
- Whiz up a nutritious and yummy smoothie
- Relax with a cup of tea
- Watch a show on Netflix
- Enjoy a session with your foam roller
- Tune into your favorite podcast
- Enjoy a quiet and relaxing post workout stretch

I also hand out larger rewards now and then. I might tell myself that after completing my four-week online work-out program, I can treat myself to a spa pedicure. I may have been planning to book that pre-summer pedicure anyway, but it is nice to tie it into sticking to my goals. It makes the trip to the spa feel a tad more sumptuous.

I've also turned this whole tactic upside down and approached the situation with a completely opposite mind-set. I'm at a point in my health and fitness journey where the activity itself is the reward. As I mentioned in chapter 8, running is my friend! I look forward to my runs and view them as much needed me time. They give me energy. They allow me to enjoy a dose of fresh air and sunshine. They give me time and space to work through my thoughts. They provide a private venue to listen to somewhat ridiculous music. (I've tuned into the eighties lately with *Wham!* running on my playlist.) So even though there are moments during my workouts that feel hard, they still classify as dreamy to me. I think to myself, if you push yourself to get out of this warm snuggly bed (challenge), you get to hit the road with your tunes and feel energized (reward)! A lot of motivation is about the perspective you choose to take.

If you are someone who dreads or avoids physical exercise, you might find this change in mindset effective. I will be the first to admit, back when I first started running, this approach was challenging for me. As someone new to running, I frankly found the entire experience painful, and was usually counting down the minutes for it to end. Once I pushed past the initial week or two of discomfort, I found I looked forward to the runs. At that particular time in my life, I was running with a partner. My chats with her became part of the reward.

Ask yourself if there is any part of your workout that feels like a reward. Do you like the music they play in your fitness class? Do you enjoy wearing your cute little workout outfit? Do you have a workout buddy you like spending time with? Finding even a small sliver of reward in your activity can be very helpful in shifting your mindset.

Although I rarely lack motivation to exercise, I'm a bit less reliable when it comes to another area of self-improvement I am working on. For the past few years, I have been trying to adopt a committed, consistent meditation practice. I think I struggle because I am someone who likes to keep moving. Settling down to sit and just be is definitely challenging for me, which obviously is a clear sign meditation is exactly what I need!

I have tried a few of my own motivation tactics, and I do find them helpful. I have penciled meditation in right after getting the kids off to school. I tell myself that once I get the hectic part of the morning behind me (practical task), I get to indulge in me time and sit in a state of calm, quiet solitude (dreamy task). After nagging the kids to get out of bed and throwing lunches together, the morning meditation session takes on a dreamy tone for sure!

Aim to Impress

I am a big believer that inspiration and motivation are more effective if they come from within. The choices I make each day are fueled by my inner desires and the vision of my healthiest self. I'm really only looking to impress myself, and am not concerned with what other people think; with one exception (or rather two).

As a mother of two, I am keenly aware that I am being watched. The lifestyle choices I make don't just impact my own personal health, their effects trickle into the psyche of my children. I am motivated to set a good example for my kids. I want them to witness first-hand the benefits of good nutrition and an active lifestyle. I want them to put what they learn into action, and live long, healthy and happy lives themselves!

I can't help but feel a bit of satisfaction when I notice my children picking up on my cues. As the only female in our family, I don't always connect with our household's popular interests and hobbies. I can't keep up on the extreme mountain bike trails, and I struggle to get excited about engines, drones and power tools. Imagine my delight recently when my fourteen year old suddenly took a keen interest in one of *my* hobbies, lifting weights! I have been quietly going about my workouts for their entire lives, and I'm now seeing my example rub off. It's been a heart-warming way for the two of us to connect. I helped him design a little routine, and walked him through how to use proper form. I'm also told I make the best post-workout smoothies!

Even if your children aren't tagging along with you on your runs, or jumping to join you at the pool, I encourage you to continue modeling your healthy habits. You never know when you might get a little tap on your shoulder, asking for an invitation to join!

When it comes to food, our kids are joining us around the dinner table, so the impact of our choices is more direct. It actually amazes me just how significantly our modelling impacts our children's food choices.

My husband quit drinking alcohol a couple of years ago in an effort to adopt a healthier lifestyle. Before that time, he frequently reached for a beer or cocktail when settling in to watch a hockey game with the boys. One of our sons felt the need to be "just like Daddy", and insisted on concocting his own special drink each game night. This was usually some kind of mocktail he formulated out of sparkling water, juice and cherries. As innocent as it all sounds, there was something unsettling about it for me. I felt like the seeds were being planted; that an evening on the couch meant a drink and bowl of chips in hand. During play-off season, this habit could quickly get out of hand. When my husband quit drinking alcohol, game night snacks soon became ice water and almonds. Interestingly, the requests for "special drinks" magically just ended without a word. This small example really hit home with me, because the effects were so instant.

If you have little ones in your life, (children, grandchildren, nieces, nephews, friends) why not tap into the motivation to impress them! Modelling healthy habits will result in a win-win situation.

Set Mini Goals

While I prefer to think long-term when considering my lifestyle choices, I do tap into mini goals that I set for myself to spark a bit of excitement and enthusiasm. Every now and then I come up with a particular area of interest that I want to explore. Last year I decided to improve my posture and my physical poise. I have always admired the grace and elegance of ballet dancers, and decided it was time for me to explore my own inner-ballerina. Although I'm normally drawn to adrenaline pumping activities, I signed myself up for an online barre program. My quest to become more graceful motivated me to stick with the program, even when my reflection in the mirror was falling over or moving like a robot. After a full year of dedicated practice, I proudly feel that I am moving with more grace, fluidity and flexibility.

Do you have a mini goal in mind that could serve to ignite a bit of passion into your health routines? Maybe you have always dreamed of becoming a runner, but haven't gotten around to it. Why not set your sights on that community 5K taking place in a few months? Take the next step and actually sign yourself up! Is there an activity you did as a child that you would like to revisit? Maybe you were on the swim team in high school but haven't dipped a toe into the pool in decades. Would you like to get back in the game and improve your swimming stroke?

Identify Quick Hits

Sometimes sources of inspiration hit you when you least expect it. I encourage you to jump on these opportunities when they present themselves. It can be something as tiny as a great song on the radio! Whenever I hear a song that gets me energized, I immediately add it to my running playlist. A great tune can be a powerful tool in adding pep to your step! Next time you hear an uplifting song, be sure to make note or download it before it slips your mind.

During a cycling trip in Croatia, (with my father who was eighty one at the time) I was powering up a hill and someone called out, "Here comes the thoroughbred!" I was flattered and immediately tapped into that image. A year later, I use the thoroughbred visualization regularly to motivate and push myself forward. There is a song by Birdie called *Wild Horses* that puts me in my thoroughbred mindset, and I sometimes play it on repeat when I'm in the mood.

Have you ever had an image come to your mind that got you excited and inspired? A ballerina, a horse, a cheetah, a swan...add these images to your arsenal of uplifting and inspiring thoughts. Draw on them in those moments you wish to channel their being. It sounds a bit wonky, but it works for me!

I was hit with a little boost of interest one day while watching my son play soccer. I could not help but marvel at the fast and agile footwork of all the players. The next day on my run, I incorporated a few minutes of soccer "fast feet" on a particularly rocky stretch of the trail. I've stuck with incorporating this short moment of agility training into my fitness routine, and look forward to this segment of my run each day. (A song with a great rhythm helps.) I won't be signing up for a soccer league, but I like to think I'm setting myself up with skills that will help me as I age.

What tidbits of inspiration speak to you? What little sparks can you reach for each day to ignite a bit of passion? Music is certainly one of the best motivators! Finding catch phrases and quotes that really speak to you definitely come in handy during moments you might feel frustrated or deflated. *Beachbody* trainer Autumn Calabrese often says, "You can do anything for a minute." I've repeated this one to myself on many occasions! Gather a list of all your favorite quotes, catch phrases, songs, and inspiring images and add these to your wellness journal or Pinterest boards. Keep adding to your inventory of inspiration on a regular basis and draw on it when the mood strikes.

Seek Companionship

As an introvert, I tend to view my exercise time as an opportunity for introspection and to replenish my energy reserves. I really value this alone time in my life. I am actually motivated to seek out this solitude! Being alone with my thoughts is truly a reward, and probably gives me just as much of a boost as the increase in my heart rate.

Other people like my husband, who are more extroverted in nature, enjoy comradery and company when doing fitness activities. He is much more motivated to accomplish his goals if he has other people relying on him to show up. He also grew up playing a variety of team sports, so he tends to thrive on competition! Knowing this about himself, he chooses hockey and group bootcamp classes as some of his regular forms of exercise.

The bottom line is, get to know yourself and what drives and motivates you. If you are more likely to stay on track if you are participating in a social activity, then use this to your advantage. If you are like me and crave the alone time and escape, focus your efforts on structuring a routine that fills your needs. The great thing is that we are all individuals! The better you get to know yourself, and what makes you tick, the more easily you can set yourself up for success.

Elevating Actions and Inspiration

- Identifying strategies and techniques that keep you motivated is an important key to success. Take the time to do a bit of self-discovery to find ways to motivate yourself to stick with your health goals.

- Providing yourself with regular mini rewards can be very effective at helping you stay on track with your plans. Dream up a list of small rewards you can indulge in after completing a difficult task. They should be small, accessible and ideally free! They will serve as little bright spots to look forward to after a job well done.

- Consider flipping your mindset by viewing activity or exercise as the reward! Think about all the elevating aspects of an activity that make it enjoyable; the company you share, the music, the outdoors, the energy….etc. Focus your attention on the positive aspects of the experience to shift your mindset away from feelings of dread!

- Find motivation in the fact that you are setting a good example for the younger generation. Think about the positive impact your healthy example is having on your children, grandchildren and other little eyes that might be watching!

- Although long-term health is the ultimate goal, consider setting mini short-term goals for yourself. These small goals might inspire you to try something new, or could add a renewed sense of excitement to your current efforts.

- Keep your eyes and ears peeled for quick hits of inspiration. These might include uplifting songs, inspirational quotes or dreamy images that you can draw on now and then to push yourself. It's helpful to keep track of these in a journal so you can pull them out when needed. Have fun adding to your lists regularly, building up an inventory of quick hits!

10

CAPITALIZE ON THE SEASON AND CIRCUMSTANCES

Is there a time of year or season that ignites a sense of energy and enthusiasm in you? Perhaps there is a period of the year where motivation to focus on health and self-care feels effortless and breezy.

Maybe you are a die-hard sun seeker and thrive in warm climates. There is no need to set an alarm in the mornings. You find it easy to rise early with the sun, and look forward to your morning walks listening to the birds. Jump-starting your day with invigorating movement makes you feel vibrant and alive. The farm markets and vegetable stands are overflowing with a tantalizing array of fresh produce, so it's easy to plan and eat nutritious meals. You love the water, so you seek out any opportunity to hit the beach, enjoying refreshing swims on a regular basis through-out the week. Life feels grand when the sun is shining!

Perhaps you find yourself on the other end of the spectrum. You grew up in the mountains, and consider yourself a bit of a snow princess! The sight of the first snow-flakes of the season gives you a thrill of anticipation for the upcoming ski season ahead. You are perfectly content to bid farewell to the hot, humid summer and the mos-quitoes and blackflies. You thrive in the cold! It feels refresh-ing and exhilarating to experience the great outdoors when the mercury drops. After a day on the slopes, you love coming home to unwind with a nourishing bowl of hearty vegetable stew, a warm bath and a good book. As a home-body, you are in your element during this time of year! Winter gives you a sense of peace and calm and an oppor-tunity to focus inward.

Seek out That Silver Lining

Most of us probably fall somewhere in the middle. I think the key is to try to find the silver lining in *every* season, and seek out opportunities to enhance your health, instead of focusing on the roadblocks and challenges.

I've given this topic a lot of thought, as I am one of those people whose mood and energy levels go up and down with the seasons. The spring and winter in Nova Scotia where I live can be particularly challenging times of the year for me. I sometimes find myself frustrated and unmotivated when the weather doesn't cooperate with my plans. I thrive in the summer and fall, when the weather suits the outdoor activities I enjoy the most, such as runn-ing, hiking and cycling. I came to the realization that in order to thrive in a state of health and wellbeing all twelve months of the year, I needed to develop some strategies to approach the more challenging seasons with a different mindset.

Do you also find that sour and glum thoughts creep in when a certain season approaches? What if you challenged yourself to identify the hidden gems of opportunity that your least favorite time of year has tucked away? Instead of just accepting things as they are, why not seek inspiration in the perceived roadblocks? Embrace the situation and find joy in the opportunity to increase the variety in your life.

I came to the realization that the icy sidewalk conditions that were hampering my running efforts provided me with the perfect "excuse" to change up my routine. Our bodies grow accustomed to the same type of activity on repeat. For me, this sometimes means getting stuck on a plateau, or overusing certain body parts, leading to injury. Tapering down my running routine, and focusing my efforts on something new and challenging, turned out to be just what my mind and body were craving. By being forced to take some of my activity inside, I was able to really focus my attention on the barre and yoga programs I was interested in. By working on my core strength and flexibility for a change, I was left feeling more balanced, and in a better state of overall physical health.

Perhaps it is not ice and snow that have you stuck inside, but rather scorching heat and humidity. I realize that many people live in locations where heat is actually a hindering factor. Maybe the summer heat means that you also need to change things up and take your activity inside, where the comfort of the air conditioning keeps you motivated and moving.

Have you considered that the hotter periods of the year present an opportunity to refresh and revisit your schedule and infuse it with some variety? You could switch your outdoor activities to early morning or late evening when the temperatures are a bit cooler. On a trip to Barbados several years ago, I noticed that the locals tended to participate in a lot of outdoor fitness classes in the evenings. The sun sets quite early in Barbados year round, (between 5:30 and 6:30 p.m.) so these outdoor classes take place in the dark. Although I'm accustomed to being active during daylight hours, their choice to get out and active after dark made perfect sense for the environment they live in.

If you find yourself in the position that the weather is cramping your style, why not go with the flow? Accept what you can't change, and look for new and creative ideas to explore. You might be pleasantly surprised by the discovery of a new activity. A change in your daily schedule might just provide a boost of interest and energy.

Connect With Your Inner Child

As I child, I loved and looked forward to the winter season. I grew up in northern New Brunswick where the winters were long, cold and snowy! The blanket of snow and the frigid temperatures opened up opportunities to engage in so many of my favorite activities that were only available during this very special time of year. Our tiny village maintained an outdoor ice rink that was at the end of my street. It was fun, easy and convenient to lace up my skates regularly. I also lived fifteen minutes away from a very small ski hill. As tiny as it was, it was a wonderful way to spend the day with my friends as a teen, getting fresh air and exercise while spying on our latest crush on the chairlift. Family outings during my childhood included snowshoeing in the woods behind our home (with hot chocolate breaks under the snow laden trees).

I have such fond winter memories from my child-hood, that it caused me to pause and reconsider the downer perspective I adopted in my adulthood. My attitude towards winter had taken on such a negative tone! Once the excitement and festivities of the holidays died down, I found it challenging to remain motivated, optimistic and energized when it was so darn cold out!

I decided to tap into that child-like wonder I possessed in the past. Although skiing and skating are not as easily accessible to me right now, I live in a rural area with an abundance of trails at my doorstep. The past few winters I have really embraced winter hiking. We don't have enough snow to require snowshoes in these parts, but I feel a connection to my past each time I set foot on the wintry trails. I found I actually enjoy winter hiking more than any other season! The forest has a magical quality in the winter that is not present other times of the year. I particularly appreciate admiring the animal tracks and trails in the snow. I can safely say I did not miss one daily "woodsy walk" this past winter. Having my little dog Coco staring at me by the door with puppy dog eyes certainly helped get me out the door each day. That being said, those walks were the highlight of my days, and I am missing the snow and cold weather now that the black flies and ticks are back in season!

If you find yourself stuck in a rut and lamenting the weather, try reconnecting with your inner child. Did you have a different perspective on things back when life seemed more fun and full of adventure? What seasonal activities did you adore in your childhood that you haven't attempted in years? Did you enjoy sliding in the snow or skating? When was the last time you tried these outdoor activities as an adult? Did you spend summer days at the lake? When was the last time you took a refreshing dip and reconnected with your love of swimming? It really is a fun exercise to do a bit of reminiscing. It may just ignite a spark of enthusiasm for an old passion and set you off on a new path towards better health.

Seek Out Win-Win Situations

Look for creative ways to fit in a little extra exercise! Each season offers a unique opportunity to combine physical activity and household tasks. Raking leaves, mowing the lawn, washing windows, weeding the flower beds, shoveling snow…these are all fantastic forms of exercise.

I have learned to seek out and savour these win-win situations as they arise each season. I actually find that I *enjoy* shovelling snow because it reminds me of fort building as a child! Piling firewood also brings back fond memories of working alongside my father. Helping him stock our basement with firewood was a fall tradition I looked forward to each year. (We heated our home with a wood furnace back then. It guzzled a hefty seven cords of wood each winter!)

What if you reframed a few seasonal tasks and challenged yourself to appreciate them on a whole new level? Would scraping the ice and snow off your windshield feel more appealing if you viewed it as a chance to keep your arms strong? While weeding your flower garden, you could choose to enjoy the beauty of the blooms, but also the opportunity to move and stretch your body.

Milk it While You Can

This next tidbit of advice goes without saying, but I think it is a good reminder to make hay while the sun shines! When the page of the calendar turns, and it just happens to be "the most wonderful time of the year" for you, milk it all you can! Revel in the fact that you can engage in some of your favorite outdoor activities, and take full advantage of the opportunity. Don't let the days slip by with obligations and endless to do lists that keep you from enjoying some of your favorite healthy activities.

As soon as the weather warms up enough in these parts, I have my bicycle tuned and ready to go. The cycling season is fairly short for me, so I take full advantage of this favorite activity whenever I can. These days I am up and out the door pedaling at 5:30 a.m. (I like to avoid the traffic!) It feels delicious to start my day doing something that brings me so much joy. I think I appreciate it even more knowing that I can't do it all year round.

When your favorite fruits and veggies are in season, indulge in them as much as possible. They truly are the tastiest during their peak season, and should be savoured and enjoyed to their full potential. Anyone who knows me personally is aware of my blueberry obsession. I eat them all year round, as I always have some tucked away in my freezer. When blueberry season hits, I really up my game! With my faithful companion and blueberry picker extraordinaire in tow (my mom), I usually haul in at least forty pounds at the u-pick every August. My family gobbles these fresh treats up fast and furiously. I have been known to incorporate blueberries into every meal of my day (snacks included). Of course, it's a bonus that blueberries are considered to be a super food by many! It's a winning combination.

As I mentioned in chapter 4, go the extra step and pencil yourself in. Don't let your favorite season fizzle away without doing (and eating) all those things that bring you so much joy. If you want to do more skiing, this winter, go ahead and pre-purchase a set of passes. (It usually makes economic sense anyway as they are discounted during the off-season.) If you'd love to spend more time on your bicycle, make a plan to get it to the bike shop early for a tune up, so it is rearing to go when you are. Pre-book your valuable summer weekends with the activities that are important to *you,* before they get booked up by someone else! Make a commitment to visit the farmers' markets on the weekend to get your pick of the freshest of produce.

Elevating Actions and Inspiration

- If there is a particular time of year you often find yourself feeling deflated and unmotivated, try to seek out the silver lining. Put some thought into how you could change things up to spark some interest and energy. If you are forced to take your exercise routine inside, try to appreciate the change of pace and scenery. Try out something new like an online fitness, yoga or dance class or lifting weights.

- Revisit your daily schedule and look for ways to fit in activity that complements the weather. An early morning or late evening session might better suit the temperature outside.

- It's always helpful to tap into your inner-child when you find yourself feeling uninspired. Try looking at a situation with a sense of childhood awe. Are there activities that you enjoyed immensely in the past that would feel invigorating to revisit?

- Seek out win-win situations that each unique season has to offer. Enjoy the opportunity to fit in extra physical activity while simultaneously crossing household tasks off your to do list!

- Be sure to take advantage of your favorite time of year and pack in as much goodness as possible! Make a commitment to yourself that you will prioritize participating in all the outdoor activities of the season that truly bring you joy.

- Go out of your way to enjoy the healthy seasonal foods when they are at their very best.

11

DRESS FOR SUCCESS

In my book, *Elevate Your Personal Style*, I discuss the importance of putting your best foot forward each day by dressing and presenting yourself in a manner that makes you feel happy, confident and pulled together. Although it sounds superficial at first glance, what we wear actually has a significant impact on the energy we bring to our days, and how feel on the inside.

After leaving my corporate accounting career to stay home and raise my children, I spent many years slopping around my house in less than flattering attire. I couldn't see the point in bothering to focus on how I looked, because my days were spent changing diapers, wiping snotty noses and mopping up spills. When I finally made the decision to start nurturing my personal appearance and image, I noticed a shift in my energy. An upgrade to both my mindset and wardrobe had a dramatic and transformative effect on my sense of self-worth and overall enthusiasm for life.

This concept applies to each and every moment of your day! Dressing and presenting yourself in a pleasing manner is not reserved for those times you venture out into the public world. That's because the root of your intentions should not focus on pleasing others, but rather pleasing yourself. Putting deliberate thought and effort into your sartorial choices impacts your mood and mindset, no matter what activity you are engaging in; cleaning the house, meeting clients at the office, snuggling up for a Friday night movie, enjoying a yoga class, or pounding the pavement on your morning run. Yes, what you wear when you are enjoying exercise and active pursuits is important too!

There is no doubt that charging into an important business meeting in a power suit is going to boost your confidence. At the onset of my accounting career, my role as the lead field auditor often called for my participation in audit committee meetings. As a fledgling accountant, the atmosphere in these boardrooms was extremely intimidating. I viewed my business suits as a coat of armor! Dressing for success in these situations definitely played a role in elevating my confidence and composure.

The same holds true for how you approach dressing for your workouts. If you show up wearing ill-fitting, sloppy and threadbare attire, it's likely you will enter your workouts with a mindset and attitude that matches it; one that feels heavy, tired, burdensome and sluggish. Making the choice to wear something fun, pretty, flattering and inspiring will have the opposite effect. If you feel good in your clothes, you will approach the task at hand with more positivity and passion. This option sounds a lot more uplifting, and will certainly produce better results.

I'm not suggesting that we all work out dressed in designer activewear, with a full face of makeup painted on! Obviously, the term activewear implies that the gear is destined to endure some abuse. (Note: If you aren't sweating in it, you might not actually be working out!) I'm simply pointing out that having a pleasing and pretty collection of exercise clothes that is in good condition can elevate your fitness experience. Clothing that feels good to put on might give you that extra little boost you need to get out of bed and show up, run an extra mile, or hold a pose and extra few seconds.

Two years ago, my father took me on a cycling trip to Croatia to celebrate his eighty first birthday. The tour included accommodations on a boat with a group of travelers from around the globe. It's always fun to meet and observe how people from other countries and cultures approach life. Of course, being a Francophile, I gravitated towards a woman named Sabine from France. I jumped at any opportunity to chat with her, and enjoyed exchanging thoughts and opinions on a wide range of topics including food, travel, the environment and aging. I also quietly observed and made note of her cycling fashion choices each day! We were averaging fifty to sixty kilometers a day in extremely hilly terrain (in the heat!)

Although this was no place to make a fashion statement, Sabine still managed to do so! She always wore the cutest of coordinated cycling outfits that matched her friendly personality. Despite the smearing of sweat and sunscreen on her face, I noticed she had made the effort to apply a flattering and delicate touch of eyeliner each day! She exuded vitality and style, even while huffing and puffing up the steepest of hills!

Take an Inventory

What is the state of your workout wear? Athletic clothing is often overlooked as part of our overall wardrobes. Set aside a bit of time to dump it all on the bed and perform an assessment of your collection. Is there anything in there that is definitely operating well past its best before date? Items with frayed elastics, stretched out waistbands and peek holes in unflattering locations should definitely be tossed. I also find that after a certain amount of time and wear, the smell of perspiration gets baked in so deeply, that it is impossible to get out (even with special detergents and vinegar rinses). Once my kids start making comments about the offensive odor emanating from one of my freshly laundered shirts, I know it's time to toss it.

Upgrade with Inspiring Pieces

The next time you have the need and budget for new athletic clothing, pick up something that really catches your attention and makes you smile. Workout wear is an area of your wardrobe that can be fun to play around with and explore a different side of your personality. While I normally dress in a very neutral color palette, I enjoy adding a bit of sparkle and color to my fitness attire. Printed tights, sparkly headbands, flashy running shoes…. the sky is the limit! Dressing for your workouts can be a form of self-expression! This past year my obsession with barre workouts led me to treat myself to a cute little leotard. I can now play ballerina in my basement! (I got the exact one I always pined for as a little girl.) It might sound silly, but it is fun to wear and elevates the experience of my daily workouts.

Prioritize Your Purchases

You don't need to spend a fortune on workout clothing and gear. The truth is, if you are using it for its intended purpose, it isn't going to last forever! I prioritize which items I am willing to drop a bit more cash on, and look for deals on the others. Since I run almost every single day, comfortable tights with a secure side pocket for my phone are high on my list. I am a die-hard fan of Lululemon's offerings, which are certainly on the pricey end of the spectrum. I pick up tank tops, bras, shirts and socks for discounted prices at a Canadian store called Winners (TJ Maxx being the American equivalent).

Don't Skimp on the Important Stuff

Certain items in your fitness arsenal are more important than others, depending on the types of activities you participate in. I've learned that there are certain scenarios where "bootstrapping" it doesn't pay off. Are there pieces of your fitness gear or clothing that aren't performing? Could upgrading or replacing them have a positive impact on your fitness endeavors?

During the summer of 1996, my father and I embarked on a cross-Canada cycling trip. We were not seasoned cyclists, and I definitely made a few errors in judgement during the packing process. Would you believe that I packed jean shorts? Yes, I intended to cycle over five thousand kilometers in a pair of cut-offs! This delusional thinking lasted one day. The first day of our adventure took us from Victoria to Vancouver, British Columbia. Upon arriving in Vancouver, we immediately upgraded our wardrobes to include nicely cushioned, moisture wicking bottoms! The jean shorts were left behind, as there was no room for them in my limited cargo space.

As a runner, comfortable and proper fitting shoes are an area I never skimp on. I have my shoes fitted at a small local retailer that offers expert advice. When it comes to athletic shoes, comfort always wins over style!

I have a friend who really inspires me with her love for and commitment to lake swimming. By investing in a good quality wetsuit, she was able to extend her swimming season well past the comfort zone of most people! She managed to maintain her weekly swimming schedule for nine months of the year – an amazing feat in Nova Scotia!

If you find yourself avoiding certain activities because certain pieces of gear just aren't living up to their promise, consider that it might be time for an upgrade. Have a look at your budget and prioritize any key items that might add to the safety and enjoyment of your activity.

Dress for the Weather

I'm a Canadian girl, born and raised. Most people I come across when travelling usually associate my home country with cold, snowy weather. They aren't far off the mark! Even though we enjoy four lovely seasons, winter seems to hold its firm grip for months on end. I therefore consider myself somewhat of an expert on dressing for winter conditions! I'm one of those people who is cold-blooded, so I'm always on the hunt for ways to add a little heat and comfort to my life.

Do you also live in the type of climate that makes you want to pack it all in and hibernate for the winter? Getting active in the great outdoors can be a challenge during the bitter and harsh months of winter. That being said, I'm a big fan of getting outside each day, even if it is just for a small amount of time. Natural sunlight and fresh air invigorates my soul! The key to keeping your body moving during the winter months is to take a twofold approach; take it inside, (which I discussed in Chapter 10) and dress for the weather. I draw on both of these tactics and it allows me to stick to my health and fitness goals, no matter what weather Old Man Winter throws at me.

Yes, hibernation is tempting, but embracing the situation and being smart, flexible and prepared is elevating! I run twelve months of the year, and have learned how to dress in a manner that keeps me safe and warm. If you too live in an area of the world that experiences frigid temperatures, I encourage you to keep on truckin' through the seasons and invest in the quality gear you need to do so. I own one pair of very special (yes expensive) running tights that are designed for the coldest of winter running. They are fabulous and were worth the investment in my health. Beyond those tights, I just layer up and hit the road. If the footing conditions are too icy and dangerous, I definitely take a pass and choose something indoors.

My parents have lived the "snowbird" life for over a decade. For those not familiar with this term, it refers to retirees who escape the harshest months of the year by migrating south to sunnier destinations. This past winter, the global pandemic squashed all travel plans. Instead of bunkering down and hibernating, they did their best to take advantage of the beauty of winter. One of the first things they had to do was buy some proper winter clothing!

I had fun helping my mom pick out a stylish wool camel coat for running errands. She also picked up a hip length puffer coat so she could continue with her walking in warmth and comfort. My dad approached his outfitting task with boyish enthusiasm. He bought a new parka, snow pants and boots so he could walk the wooded trails behind his home, no matter the weather. He grew up in a log cabin in the woods of northern Ontario, so he is no stranger to the harshest of winter conditions. (He even lived in a tent with his father one winter in the back woods to work the traps lines!) He says he enjoyed this past winter at home more than any of the last decade down south. Properly dressed for success, he was able to enjoy his nature walks in comfort and stay on track with his fitness goals.

Don't let the cold keep you cooped up! Invest in warm clothing and solid footwear that can keep you toasty and dry during any season. As long as the footing is safe, the technical clothing available these days allows us to venture outside for some fresh air and exercise during some of the toughest conditions. If my eighty-three-year-old dad is out there facing the cold, I figure I have no excuse!

Elevating Actions and Inspiration

- Don't forget to consider your fitness attire as part of your overall wardrobe. Pleasant, well-fitting clothes that you feel good in have the ability to elevate your mood and efforts while exercising.

- Sort through your current collection of activewear and toss anything that is past its prime or leaves you feeling flat and uninspired.

- When it comes time to upgrade your workout wear, seek out pieces that spark some enthusiasm and excitement inside you. Choose items that make you want to get out there and participate! It's a fun domain to experiment with different colors and patterns.

- Prioritize your purchases (unless money is no object!) Allocate the bulk of your hard-earned dollars where quality and comfort are extremely important. (Athletic shoes always fall into this category.) Pick up other pieces on sale or at discount stores. Tops in particular retain odor quite quickly, so they aren't going to last forever. It's not worth investing too much in them.

- Consider investing in good quality winter fitness attire if you live in a cold climate and tend fall into a trap of inactivity when the temperature drops. Choose items that are designed to perform well on the most frigid of days. Don't let the cold stop you from achieving your health and fitness goals.

12

LISTEN TO YOUR BODY

Taking action towards better health is just as often about "not doing" as it is about "doing". Knowing when to step back is as important as knowing when to step it up! Rest and recovery are vital to overall health and wellbeing, and yet in our "go, go, go" society they are often overlooked or scoffed upon.

Certainly, a go-getter attitude is advantageous when it comes to achieving health and wellness goals. Taking charge of your wellbeing, and choosing healthier options and behaviours, takes focus and dedication. Resisting the urge to hit snooze in order to fit your invigorating workout into your busy day takes commitment. Taking a pass on the greasy chips your husband is scarfing down next to you on the couch takes willpower. If you are succeeding at putting your health goals at the top of your list of priorities and staying committed to your fitness and nutrition plans, you should be proud!

Tune In To Your Body

That being said, when we are in a state of hyper-focus, it can be easy to lose sight of the big picture. I speak from experience on this one! In fact, I specifically wrote this chapter as a letter to myself. In moments of delusion and denial, I plan to reach for it and remind myself of my own wise words! I can't count the number of times I ignored blaring warning signals from my body, all in the name of sticking to a pre-set fitness schedule. (As I mentioned, the accountant in me is a sucker for ticking off boxes.) Lists and workout calendars can serve as effective tools in keeping you on track with your goals, but they should be devised with flexibility, forgiveness and kindness in mind.

Listen to your body. It sounds so simple, but I'll be the first to admit, I'm not always in tune with what it is telling me (or screaming and hollering at me). I have, on several occasions, sacrificed my own health by ignoring my body's cry for rest, recovery and patience.

We live on a rural property surrounded by an abundance of natural foliage and shrubbery. It represents a treasure trove for Christmas crafters like me! Every holiday season, I enjoy gathering festive boughs and branches to decorate our home and to share with friends. One particular year, I went a tad overboard in my zealous quest to amass the finest pile of Christmas branches ever known to man. A North Pole brain freeze is the only plausible explanation for my frenzied branch-clipping behaviour.

The next morning, I could barely move my arm or hand. I brushed the pain and numbness off as a little muscle soreness, and never gave it a second thought. After all, I was fit and strong, and could blast my way through any workout *Beachbody* could throw at me.

Ignoring the three alarm fire in my arm was a disastrous error on my part. I have since been educated on the very important distinction between "good pain" and "bad pain" by my chiropractor. Over the course of several weeks, I discounted the unrelenting pain in my forearm and elbow and carried on with the weightlifting program I was staunchly committed to completing. A month later, I couldn't even hold a glass of water in my right hand. Instead of allowing my body to rest after the repetitive strain caused by my insane pruning episode, I caused further damage. I developed a nasty case of tennis elbow that painfully stuck around for an entire year; completely sidelining all my upper body workout efforts. By ignoring my body's bellow for rest, I took twenty steps backwards!

Know Your Limits

While I am a big fan of rising to a challenge and pushing yourself a bit outside of your comfort zone, it is equally important to know your limits. Once again, I've learned this concept the hard way!

I'd love to report that my not-so-festive pruning injury taught me a lesson, but sadly I've had other less than shining moments of ignorance, denial and regret. A few years ago we booked a dream trip to the south of France. I had fairy tale visions of hiking from one medieval village to the next through valleys laden with the scent of wild rosemary. I pictured myself gracefully sauntering along cobblestone streets for hours, dipping into the odd little chic boutique to satisfy my desire to add a touch of authentic French girl style to my wardrobe. I imagined our family joyfully cycling together on winding roads under the glowing Provençal sunshine. Yes indeed, this trip was going to cross off many of my bucket list dreams.

The morning of our departure, I decided to rise early and squeeze in one last workout before tying up the loose ends of my packing. With visions of my bikini-clad body sunbathing on a French country terrace, I decided to "up my game", and put in a final strong effort with my last pre-trip workout. Ignoring the fact that I have long history of lower back injuries, I foolishly decided to bump up the weight on my one-legged squats. I reached for a twenty five pound dumbbell; a five pound bump in weight, and a significant increase for a small woman. I should have known better! My back is finicky on the best of days, and I have to be cautious and conservative when lifting.

If you have ever suffered a lower back injury, you will know what I mean when I refer to that millisecond where you are not quite sure what just happened. It's like an electric jolt through your spine that leaves you stunned, before you realize with dread that something is really not right! I fell to the floor in shock shouting, "No, no, no, no, no!" I knew things had just taken a very bad turn.

Well, there was no way this dream trip was going to happen without me, so I somehow mustered the gumption and energy to fly across the Atlantic ocean. I travelled through the airports by wheelchair, and literally crawled to my seats! (One silver lining is that we jumped all the line ups!) This was certainly not the dreamy, sparkly version of my trip to France I had concocted in my head. I spent the first two days in our villa flat on my back with ice and ibuprofen. We did end up having a lovely time, once I lowered my expectations and took it easy with our outings (au revoir hiking, cycling and manoeuvring tight dressing rooms in chic boutiques). I knew my limits, ignored them, and I paid the price!

Do a Daily Check-In

As I reflect on these stories, I really do hope that I have learned my lesson. I hope you can gain some wisdom from my foolish ways and avoid the same situations! I have made it a part of my morning routine to check-in with my physical and emotional self to determine what actions and behaviours will serve me best in the day ahead. Each morning while *sningering,* (my invented word for that delicious time of snuggling and lingering just before you actually get out of bed) I ask myself the question, "What does my body need today?" I check in on my aches and pains, and my overall sense of wellbeing. My goal is to approach the day ahead with an attitude of kindness towards myself, knowing when I need a bit of a push and motivation, and knowing when I need to back off . Like most other areas of life, it's all about finding the right balance! Your body naturally knows what it needs, so you need to tune in attentively to its whisperings.

Elevating Actions and Inspiration

- Resist the urge to soldier on with a workout plan when your body is telling you it is clearly injured, or requires a recovery break. Injuries are never worth it and will only leave you further behind from achieving your goals.

- Don't ignore your aches and pains. Dig a bit deeper and learn to identify the difference between "good pain" and "bad pain". When your body is obviously telling you it is time for a rest, sit up and listen! The world isn't going to end if you don't finish a workout, or don't tick every box this week (reminder to self).

- Know your limits and respect them! Do you have a nagging injury from days gone by that flares up every now and then? While I don't recommend dwelling on your limitations, you do need to work around them to prevent further pain, frustration and damage. Push yourself, and strive for improvement, but always within the boundaries of your limits. Stay safe!

- Check in with yourself regularly, setting aside your ego, expectations and excuses. Have an honest conversation with yourself each day to determine what actions and behaviours will serve to elevate your health!

- Adopt an attitude of gentleness towards yourself. Each morning I wake up and state, "Be kind to yourself." Saying these words out loud serves as a reminder of the outlook and tone I want to set for the day.

13

BE A BOSS OF BEDTIME

I can think of very few things in life that feel as delicious as a good night's sleep. I don't know that I *truly* appreciated the gift of uninterrupted sleep until I gave birth to my second son. It was on this momentous day that the notion of a good night's sleep, that I had taken for granted for so long, became unattainable. He is now fourteen years old and is such a joy in my life. He is thoughtful, loving, sensitive and creative. He is a sweetheart through and through, and I love him with all my heart. I wanted to preface this next statement with glowing remarks about my dear boy, because the truth is, he tormented my nights for many, many years (more than I am willing to admit, especially after reading every parenting book on the market).

My reminder to any young mothers going through the hell of sleepless nights...it will eventually work itself out. It might take longer than you'd like, but the sleepless nights will one day come to an end. At some point, I simply surrendered to my reality and tried to appreciate the joy of our time together (yes, even at 2:00 a.m.). I can still feel the soft tickle of his baby fine hair on my nose as I comforted and cuddled him on those long nights. I was tired, but I was also overflowing with love. Soaking up and appreciating these magical moments with your child can take the focus away from your feelings of exhaustion.

So, as you can imagine, now that I have the nights back to myself, I'm pretty protective of my sleep. (Selfish is another word that comes to mind!) The older I get, the more I seem to require the nourishing and healing properties of a solid night of uninterrupted sleep. I really feel off on a day that I missed out on the proper rest the night before. I still can't believe I operated for so many years in such a severe state of sleep deprivation.

Do you place getting a good night's rest at the top of your priority list? My husband used to work on his laptop into the wee hours of the morning, claiming he just wasn't one of those people who needed a solid eight hours. He thought he had special powers I guess. At the time, he was a partner with a large international accounting firm, and I think that was just the excuse he told himself. He was overworked and overwhelmed, and those long hours were his survival strategy. He ended up leaving that position to work at a locally owned firm of like-minded partners, and the shift has done wonders for his health. Now that he is going to bed at a reasonable hour, he notices a significant increase in his energy and ability to focus. He was really just telling himself a story before.

If you think you might be lacking a few hours in the sleep department, why not set yourself up for success to hit the hay a little earlier. When it comes to sleep, it's important to think in terms of both *quality* and *quantity*. Instead of just lamenting about not being able to get a good night's sleep, try to actively look for ways to deal with your issues.

Set a Reminder

We traditionally think of alarms as tools to help us wake up in the morning, but my husband has used the opposite approach. His phone plays the first few notes of a cute little lullaby at 9:00 p.m. each evening as a reminder that it's time to get his shut eye. That leaves him half an hour to get through his bedtime routine before it's lights out. This trick might come in handy if you are someone who can easily lose track of time while getting lost in a Netflix binge session!

Create a Blissful Bed

Try putting in an extra effort to make your bed a soothing and comforting place to crawl into. Making our bed each morning has the greatest impact for me. Not only does it look nicer during the day, it is much more lovely to snuggle into a pleasant, tightly made bed than to wrestle with a tangle of sheets and blankets.

Is it time to upgrade your sheets or switch them out for the season? Some people enjoy cool cotton in the summer, and snuggly flannel or fleece in the winter. Choose bedding that feels soothing and comforting against your skin and scrap the pilled or threadbare set that is due for the trash or recycling bin. I make a point of drying my sheets on the line when possible. This small extra step makes crawling under the covers on laundry days that much more heavenly. Is there anything better than the sweet smell of line-dried linens?

Create a Bedtime Routine

Create a bedtime routine that puts you in a relaxed and peaceful state. Going straight from a screen to the pillow doesn't really promote a calm and quiet mindset. I enjoy and look forward to my nightly routine. It usually includes a warm bath and taking plenty of unhurried time to wash and moisturize my face and body. I also have a nice collection of sleepwear that adds a special touch to my bedtime. It's feels good to look cute and pulled together, even if I'm just crawling under the covers. I'd much rather drift off to dreamland in my chic pair of silk pajamas than a ratty old t-shirt and boxer shorts!

My husband's routine involves unwinding by giving himself a deep muscle massage with his Theragun. (These things are really pricey, but he absolutely swears by it!)

Maybe you enjoy reading or journaling before bed, or doing a few minutes of stretching. Find something that works for you and that promotes a peaceful and relaxed mind and body.

Give Sleep Meditation a Try

Both my husband and I do something we've coined as "beditation" before falling asleep. Because I tend to have a bit of a racing mind, I use this as a tool to clear my head and focus on peaceful feelings before drifting off. We both use the app *Insight Timer*, which offers so many sleep mediations, it's almost overwhelming. I bookmarked a few favorites, including some that are simply instrumental. I particularly like those that incorporate theta wave patterns. My body and brain seem to naturally relax at the familiar sound of these favorites, and I fall asleep much more easily, and in a more peaceful state because of them.

Limit Interruptions

Limiting nighttime annoyances and interruptions is another key strategy I'm working on. As much as my sweet poodle Coco wants to sneak into our bed, he has been designated his own special spot close by in his dog bed. (It's actually so fluffy and inviting, I could probably sleep in it myself. He's a lucky pooch!) Even though he's a tiny twelve pound ball of fuzz, having him in the bed definitely adds to interrupted sleep. When we recently adopted our brand new puppy Junior, I came up with a brilliant idea! My sweet son (the poor sleeper) is in charge of the puppy at night. He is responsible to get up in the wee hours of the morning to let the little guy do his business. I'm off duty! (Is it payback time perhaps?)

My husband is a snorer. (Sorry to air your dirty laundry hon). I finally convinced him to see and ENT specialist, and he had a procedure to fix a problem relating to a broken nose from many years ago. It didn't solve the snoring completely, but it definitely improved the situation. Earplugs help as well.

Tackle Tummy Troubles

I have a very sensitive digestive system. I'm usually in for a long, sleepless night if I go against my better judgement at the dinner table. Spicy and greasy foods *never* sit well with me. While I do still indulge in them from time to time, I make sure to do so earlier in the day to allow my body time to process things. Going to bed with a tummy full of fiery food never ends well.

Are you in tune with how certain foods affect your body, and therefore your quality of sleep? When my husband gave up dairy, he noticed an opening of his airways and softer skin. This dietary change actually had a positive improvement on his snoring! Does a coffee late in the day leave you feeling jittery at bedtime? Are you comfortable falling asleep on a full stomach, or would it make more sense to move your dinner hour up to an earlier time slot?

Wake Up Gently

Of course, it almost goes without saying, keep your phone either out of the bedroom, or charging on the other side of it! If you have convinced yourself you need to have it next to your bed because you use the alarm function, think "old school" on this one! We actually purchased an alarm clock that simulates the light of the rising sun and the sound of birds. It is a really pleasant and gentle way to wake up, particularly during the short days of winter. I will never go back to those jarring phone alarms that make you want to crawl under the blankets and never resurface! Being awoken in a more natural manner improves my mood in the morning and sets me off on the right foot first thing.

Nap Guilt-Free

Let's be honest, have you ever regretted a nap? I think a lot of people feel guilty about the idea of taking a nap and associate them with being lazy. I actually find them rejuvenating and try to squeeze them in now and then when my body is feeling low. I'm not shy to nap in odd places, like while I'm sitting in the car waiting for my son's soccer practice to end. I feel much more refreshed after a fifteen minute snooze than I would if I'd spent the time scrolling my phone mindlessly. A short and sweet nap can work wonders!

Elevating Actions and Inspiration

- Are you getting enough good quality sleep? If not, consider making some changes to set you up for success in achieving your sleep goals. The restorative and healing aspects of sleep have an elevating effect on our overall health, so it's an area to prioritize!

- If you have a difficult time sticking to a firm bedtime, consider fun ways to remind yourself that it's time to turn in. Setting an alarm, or even programming your internet and WIFI to shut off at a certain time, might serve as useful tools in keeping you disciplined and on track.

- Have fun creating a bedroom atmosphere that is soothing and inviting. Taking the time to make your bed each day ensures that you are faced with a welcoming scene when it's time to crawl under the covers. It's much more enticing to slip into the comfort of a neatly made bed than a tangled and twisted mess.

- Consider shopping for new bed linens if your current ones are due for an upgrade. Frayed, thinning and pilled sheets never feel nice against the skin. Choose a fabric that feels luxurious to you. I am a fan of the feel of cool cotton sheets, but if you enjoy something silky or cozy, go for it. Some people enjoy switching their sheets to coordinate with the seasons.

- Take at least a few minutes each evening to walk yourself through the ritual of a relaxing bedtime routine. Ask yourself what would set the tone to promote a restful sleep. (Hint: Getting up to speed on the latest world news is likely not the most relaxing reading material!) You could have a bath, play relaxing music, diffuse essential oils, perform a few stretches, moisturize your hands and feet, journal or read a chapter of two of the book on your nightstand.

- Consider trying a bedtime meditation to clear your mind and deeply relax your body. There are so many to choose from, some being just a few short minutes! I really enjoy them and have even introduced them to my teens.

- Seek out ways to limit the number of interruptions during the night (or if you have infants or very small children in the house, just accept the reality and try to fit in naps whenever possible). If you have a partner that snores, invest in a quality set of earplugs and/or encourage them to investigate the cause of their snoring. Solutions do exist!

- Consider how your diet might be affecting your quality of sleep. Adjusting your menu or mealtimes might have a positive impact on bedtime!

- Allowing yourself to wake up in a gentle manner can have a huge impact on your morning mood. Consider banning the sound of jolting alarms from your life! Rising with the sun is ideal, but this is often not practical certain times of the year. Our "sunrise alarm clock" has been a gamechanger for us.
- Let go of any guilt you might feel around naps. You will never regret a refreshing nap. This is especially important if you are not getting quality sleep at night. Sneak them in when the opportunity arises. If your schedule allows for it, make quick naps a regular part of your routine.

14

NAVIGATE HOLIDAYS
WITH CONFIDENCE

These days, it seems there is always a reason to celebrate. This, of course, is fabulous news! I think it is wonderful that we seek out any opportunity to come together and celebrate a special occasion, event or holiday. (Yes, I am one of those crazy people who held a first birthday party for her puppy.)

An agenda packed with festivities and parties, however, can present a challenge to those of us who are trying to maintain a healthy lifestyle. It almost seems like every "Hallmark Moment" in life is overflowing with temptations. The stage is set to lead us astray from our healthy habits and sabotage our efforts to stay on track with wellness goals.

An overabundance of food usually takes center stage at these joyous occasions. It can be extremely difficult to navigate this turbulent sea of temptations and distractions. To top it all off, stress, anxiety and holidays often go hand-in-hand for many people. Although celebrations are often cheerful events, they can also be fraught with triggers and annoyances that can lead to emotional and mindless eating. That snippy comment from your mother-in-law, or Uncle Tim's arrogant laugh, could have you headed straight for the platter of brownies to soothe your nerves.

Straying from your goals for a day here and there isn't the issue. The problem is that these "special occasions" don't really just pop up "here and there". Yes, Christmas comes but once a year, but there is a reason to celebrate at every corner. You can easily convince yourself of a valid excuse to overindulge on a very regular basis - summer barbeques, traditional holidays, birthday parties, date nights, graduations, baby showers, weddings, ...it is a never-ending list. I'm not complaining about the abundance of celebrations, but rather the excess of unhealthy food that usually goes along with them.

Just because it is a "special day" or the holiday season, doesn't mean you need to toss the healthy mindset out the window completely. It is possible to enjoy a special occasion and the treats it has to offer, without going overboard and abandoning your health goals.

Create a Vision

I encourage you to enter holidays and celebrations with a defined intention. Take the time beforehand to create a vision of how you want to celebrate the special occasion. Define your priorities.

How do you want to feel that day? What behaviours will help you achieve this state? Maybe your goal is to feel calm, happy and comfortable. You want to feel relaxed in both body and mind. This will allow you to connect meaningfully with your loved ones and really soak in the experience of the occasion. Is overdoing it on booze and rich foods going to help you achieve your vision? Is feeling dopey, bloated and uncomfortable going to put you in a state where you feel present and content? What if instead, you enjoyed a reasonable amount of food and drink, making sure to savour each bite of your holiday favorites. Instead of parking yourself next to the table of appetizers, find a cozy corner to have a one-on-one conversation with someone special.

Go the extra step and write down your thoughts. Before you head out the door, find a quiet moment to revisit your notes and remind yourself of your priorities and goals. It's so easy to glaze-over at the sight of all the decadent offerings at an event. By writing a script for yourself ahead of time, you will have something to mentally refer to when faced with temptations.

Bring Along a Healthy Option

Many celebrations come together as a group effort, with everyone pitching in to help out with the food preparations. These situations represent a great opportunity for you to ensure there are some health-friendly options on the buffet table! I love bringing colorful and enticing salads to potlucks events. Even though I might indulge in some of the more decadent offerings, I always dig into my own salad and load up my plate with a hefty serving of veggies. A classic veggies and dip tray (I usually use homemade hummus) is another favorite bring-along item. This gives you a healthy option to nibble on at events where the food centers around hors d'oeuvres and appetizers.

Healthy doesn't have to look boring! What child doesn't squeal at the sight of a heaping plate of bright pink watermelon? You can choose to keep it simple, or add a fancy touch to your presentation. I've seen some very impressive and tantalizing creations made from fruits and veggies alone! When my sister was a teen, one of her hobbies was what I would call "artistic food preparation". She was even hired by a local caterer to assist with buffet displays! She used to design the most beautiful fruit trays and salads. I'll never forget her little apple swans! My guess is, the more attractive your display, the more likely people (yourself included) will want to reach for your healthy options. It's a win-win situation for everybody!

Don't Show Up Famished

Don't deprive yourself during the hours leading up to a special event, so that you hit the buffet table in a famished and frenzied state. This spells disaster. No doubt, you will overindulge and end up feeling bloated and uncomfortable; not at all the vision you had in your mind!

Focus on eating light but nourishing meals throughout the day, knowing without guilt that you will indulge in a few special treats later on. I always make sure I have a satisfying little snack before I attend an event. This might be an apple with peanut butter, or some whole-grain crackers topped with a bit of hummus.

Focus on Your Favorites

There is no denying, one of the most pleasurable aspects of holidays is the food! We all look forward to special treats and indulgences that often only make an appearance once a year. I believe strongly that a healthy eating plan absolutely includes such treats! Food is one of life's great pleasures. There is no need to deprive yourself of the joy food has to offer. I think the key to striking a healthy balance is to check in with yourself and approach treat food in a mindful manner.

My attitude when it comes to holiday treats is to focus on my favorites. I get picky! Instead of indulging in everything and anything, I pick and choose those items that are really special to me. My mother's Christmas trifle is top on my list, and even though I consider myself a plant-based eater, I enjoy and savour every single bite of whipped cream and silky custard. I wouldn't for a second consider taking a pass on her heartwarming dessert. That being said, I'm quick to decline on the box of chocolates that gets passed around after dinner. I don't particularly like them, so why bother? Besides, I already indulged in the trifle, and I feel truly satisfied.

Approach the dessert table with a discerning eye. Do you really need to load your plate with a sample of every item on display? Do you even like lemon meringue pie? Reach instead for the pumpkin pie and reasonably sized brownie, and relish every scrumptious bite!

Plate It

If you want to stick to your health goals, while still enjoying the festive food being offered at an event, I encourage you to grab a plate. A plate sets boundaries. It allows you to both plan and measure how much food you want to consume. It's so easy to go overboard if you park yourself beside the buffet table and start nibbling away mindlessly. While you are chatting it up with Aunt Sylvia, you may not have even noticed that you just stuffed half the cheeseball down your throat (along with two dozen greasy crackers). Decide ahead of time how much is a reasonable amount of food to consume. Once you have reached your limit, step back and soak in the festivities, good company and celebratory atmosphere.

Shake Up Traditions

Traditions come and go. Just because something has been done one way for the last twenty years, doesn't mean it is set in stone. Don't be shy to shake things up and introduce new ideas and approaches that lean towards healthier behaviours.

Have fun exploring new recipes! Try substituting that old-standby dish with a lighter and healthier version. Pumpkin pie always makes a reliable appearance at our family's Thanksgiving table. A few years ago, I decided to try my hand at creating a vegan version of this favorite dessert. (Both options were still offered. I was just curious to see how my healthier version would fair in the taste test.) It was a huge hit! In fact, the following year it was specifically requested by all the non-vegans in the family. While my new pumpkin pie is still a treat, its oatmeal/pecan crust is definitely healthier than traditional pie crust made with white flour and shortening or lard.

I don't know about you, but by the time New Year's rolls around, I'm completely "holidayed out". I'm sick of all the excess and am craving simplicity and normalcy. The thought of sitting down to another heavy dinner is unappetizing. A few years ago, I hosted my parents and sister's family over for a luncheon in celebration of the New Year. New Year's feasts from the past would have served up heaping plates of roast beef, mashed potatoes and gravy. I decided to break tradition and center my menu around a theme of nourishing, heathy foods. I guess I viewed it as a cleanse after all the indulgences. I served a simple lentil soup, crusty wholegrain bread, and a festive looking salad topped with purple cabbage, blood orange slices and pomegranate seeds. The meal was capped off with fruit salad for dessert. No one complained of the lack of "treats". I think we probably just felt a sense of relief to eat delicious healthy food and to walk away from a meal feeling full and satisfied, instead of bloated and uncomfortable.

I encourage you to get creative and think outside the box when it comes to holiday traditions. Look for options and ideas that promote good health, which is really one of the best gifts you can give yourself and others you care about.

Stock Up

With two hungry teen boys in the house, our family burns through food very quickly. Things tend to ramp up even more during the holidays with everyone home from school and work. Most of you in similar situations are probably well acquainted with gargantuan holiday grocery runs!

Instead of filling your cart with chips, why not reach for healthier snack foods in the grocery aisle. Set yourself up for success! With nutritious nibbles conveniently on hand, you will be more likely to make wise choices when you get the munchies (bonus: so will the rest of your family!) Pre-made veggie trays are convenient to have in the fridge for anyone to help themselves to. I love buying a couple of large crates of clementines during the holiday season as they make a quick, sweet and satisfying snack. Pair your annual viewing of *National Lampoon's Christmas Vacation* with some crunchy carrots and hummus instead of a heaping bowl of buttery popcorn. The more healthy choices you have on hand, and the easier they are to access, the better your chances of success.

Don't Forget to Move

Just because it is a special occasion, doesn't mean you *must* take a day off from your exercise regimen. It's really about asking yourself what would serve to elevate the experience of your day. If time off to rest and relax is what your body needs, then go for it! If on the other hand, an invigorating burst of activity would clear your mind and allow you to feel more present, than choose that option.

I make a point of going for a run on Christmas day. Instead of hitting the road at the crack of dawn like I normally do, I save my run for mid to late afternoon. I don't want my exercise plans to infringe on being fully present for the gift opening with my family on Christmas morning, but I also don't want to give it up. I sneak in my run during that "afternoon slump". It's the perfect cure for a case of cabin fever, and also gives my introverted self a little break from all the commotion around me.

Why not add a family walk to your holiday traditions? If you crave that break from others that I do, sneak off by yourself for a moment of solitude.

Elevating Actions and Inspiration

- Remind yourself that it is still possible to stick to your health goals, while still enjoying the food and festivities of holidays and special occasions.

- Walk into parties and celebrations with a plan and a clear vision of how you want to show up. Write down your thoughts and read them over before you leave the house. Ask yourself how you want to feel and behave at the event, and what actions will lead you to your goal.

- Sign yourself up to make a healthy contribution to the celebration. Volunteer to bring a salad, veggie tray or wholesome casserole. Don't be shy to load your plate up with your own tasty and nutritious offering.

- Nourish yourself with a healthy snack before you attend an event where you know an excess of food will be offered. Walking into such an event in a famished state will likely lead to overeating (and a sore tummy later!)

- Exercise your right to be picky and choosy! Take a pass on mindless nibbling. Identify those festive favorites you look forward to each year, indulge and enjoy!

- Never approach a buffet table empty handed! Use a plate to keep you on track with the amount of food you consume and to avoid mindless, excessive nibbling.

- Shake up traditions by seeking out healthier versions of conventional recipes. Revisit menus from the past and consider changing things up. Sometimes a fresh approach is a welcome change for everyone – even those who are not health enthusiasts.

- Keep your pantry and fridge stocked up with healthy snack choices. Having nutritious and convenient options on hand during the busy holiday season will lead to better decision making when the munchies hit.

- Consider including physical activity as part of your holiday celebrations. Its elevating effects on your mind and body will enhance your experience of the celebrations. You can approach the rest of your day with more energy and a clearer mind.

15

GET IN TOUCH WITH THE INTANGIBLE

So much of this book has focused on what we might consider the tangible aspects of a healthy lifestyle. These are the first things that often come to mind when we are looking for ways to upgrade our health. When embarking on a journey to improve one's health, most people tend to focus their efforts on eating well and including physical activity into their schedules. This makes perfect sense, as they are important places to focus our attention. They both have such a huge impact on our wellbeing!

The term "good health" has a very broad definition and encompasses so many facets of our lives. As we all know, how we feel on the inside impacts how we feel on the outside, and vice versa. Our physical and mental health are so interconnected, that it doesn't really make sense to view them as two separate things.

Exploring some of the more intangible facets of wellness is really just as important as what foods we choose to nourish our body with and how often we get our heart pumping. I certainly don't have any background in psychology or mental health. I can only speak from experience, and share my thoughts on methods I've used personally to reduce my stress levels and improve my overall sense of happiness and contentment.

In fact, my desire to elevate my general mood each day was the inspiration behind my first self-published book, *Elevate the Everyday: Actions and Ideas to Enhance the Experience of Daily Life*. Writing this collection of short essays allowed me to do some soul-searching and learn more about myself. This permitted me to pinpoint what brings a sense of joyful contentment to my life. Of course, you don't have to write a book to do this for yourself! Why not devise your own personalized list of elevating actions that are tailored to your personality and lifestyle (your very own table of contents)! To get you started, here are a few approaches I have taken to promote a better state of mental health and overall wellness.

Clear the Less Obvious Clutter

As modern life gets busier, more and more of us are seeking out ways to simplify our lives. It's no wonder decluttering has become all the rage! People are drawn to the concept of simplicity for a reason. Clearing the clutter from our lives can have a huge impact on our mental health. People are searching for more connection, and removing meaningless things from our homes, schedules and minds allows us to focus on what is important to us.

Like so many others, I jumped on the decluttering wagon and went through my house with a fine toothed comb. An organized and streamlined home environment definitely allows me to walk through life with a greater sense of peace and calm. I quickly realized, however, that I had to expand my scope and look beyond my physical belongings.

Interestingly, when I took a step back and considered where I was investing time, I noticed there were a number of much less obvious commitments in my life that needed to be re-evaluated. Honestly, some of my insights shocked me and felt uncomfortable to admit. These were aspects of my life that brought me a great deal of joy at one point, and at first glance would be considered very healthy, soul-feeding pursuits. I learned that it is easy to get caught up in the idea or vision associated with something in your life, and forget to ask yourself if it remains a priority.

For many years, I created a lifestyle for myself that centered around my dream of owning a hobby farm. It started with a little flock of chickens, then ducks. I planted a small garden, which eventually turned into a giant vegetable plot, complete with hoop tunnels so I could grow greens straight into early winter. I then added two sheep, and then two more on top of that!

Although the animals and the homegrown food were in theory supposed to be nourishing both my body and soul, at some point it all just became too much. As my two boys grew older, they became more involved in extra-curricular activities. I was spending a lot of time catering to their needs, and had less time to focus on the "homestead". I had too many plates spinning, and found myself starting to resent all the tasks that had initially brought me joy. The breaking point was the winter we ran out of hay, and I was scrambling to figure out a solution for the sheep. I realized that this "perfect" farm life I had created wasn't something I even wanted anymore. With a heavy heart, I re-homed my feathered friends and sweet sheep to a little fibre farm (with lovely green pastures, something I could not give them in our scrubby coastal environment). I let the garden grow over with weeds and purchased all my veggies instead. I shut the whole beautiful thing down… and I felt so incredibly free.

I was actually surprised that there was not a greater sense of loss or disappointment in myself. After all, we've all been told to declutter the garage or basement, but I had not heard any suggestions to purge the healthy vegetable garden from one's life! Sometimes it's really about letting go of all the things we think we *should* keep.

Are you living the life you genuinely want right now, or is it based on a vision of what you think you *should* want? The lifestyle that suited a past season of your life might no longer be relevant, and that's perfectly okay!

The hobby farm was rewarding when the kids were tiny and I was home all the time, but became a burden as priorities changed. I don't regret all the adventures we had and the skills I learned, I was simply ready to move on. I have the memories to hold on to, which don't carry any weight at all. (I had family Christmas stockings made with our sheep's wool, which are lovely keepsakes.)

After I cleared the decks of all these obligations, I sat with the quiet for a few years. I was really hesitant to take on any new hobbies and wanted to take my time figuring out a new vision. Ultimately, this newly created sense of freedom and simplicity lead me down the path towards writing books!

While cleaning out our closets and tackling those shoeboxes of old photos can have an uplifting effect, sometimes it's the less tangible things, the ones right in front of our noses, that are harder to spot. I really encourage you to go through the exercise of contemplating all areas of your life, even the ones that you supposedly love (or think you should). Freeing up time and space from something you have grown tired of could open a door of opportunity for you. This is a great time to pull out that wellness journal and take an inventory of your life. Outside of your work and family commitments, where are you spending most of your free time? Do your interests and hobbies still align with your current goals and dreams?

Clear the Mental Clutter

While I found it rather easy to declutter the physical contents of my home and my unwanted commitments in life, the jam-packed state of my mind represented a much greater challenge.

I am a naturally anxious person, who has a tendency to ruminate and overthink things. While my analytical mind is an asset in many circumstances, (I am an accountant after all) it can also create a heavy burden on my mental health.

When it comes to setting a health goal and sticking to it, I do exceptionally well in the nutrition and fitness department. Healthy eating and regular physical activity have been a focus in my life for so long, I don't need to work very hard to convince myself of their benefits! After all the reading and research I've done on meditation and mindfulness, it's pretty clear that an anxious person like me could benefit from it greatly (actually all of us could, anxious or not).

Why, oh why, is it so hard for me to take the same approach, and stick to my commitments, when it comes to working on my inner calm? I have started and stopped a meditation routine a zillion times. As soon as I find myself in a groove with a daily practice, something rocks my boat and I'm once again drifting aimlessly. My latest excuse is that we are currently in lockdown because of the pandemic, and the kids are schooling at home. For some reason, I have decided that this prevents me from finding twenty minutes of time to myself to quietly sit and be present. This is, of course, a ridiculous way of thinking. At least I'm able to recognize that this is delusional self-talk, and I am simply trying to fool myself out of something that feels uncomfortable for me. I'm finding time to write this book! I'm finding time to walk the dog! Let's be honest, I'm finding time to scroll Instagram.

Do you share in my struggle? Have you heard all the magical and wonderful benefits of meditation, but still find it a challenge to make it a part of your life? Because this type of thing does not come easily to me, I decided to tap into some of the strategies I have used to inspire myself in other areas of wellness, and incorporate them into this habit.

- Creating visual inspiration really helps keep me on track with my goals and serves as a pleasant reminder of all the benefits available to me. I made a Pinterest board I labeled "mindfulness" that I can refer to when I need a little pick me up. All the photos give off a Zen vibe that captures the feeling of peace and acceptance I'm striving for.
- I signed up for a thirty day meditation course with an online teacher I found on the *Insight Timer* app. Her name is Fleur Chambers, and she is the woman behind the website www.thehappyhabit.com.au. In this case, having the structure of a month long program helps me stay focused. Everything is laid out for me and all I have to do is hit play!

- I got my son set up with a laptop in his bedroom for his online schooling so I could have my "home office" back to myself. I call it my office, but it's really more of a dreamy little nook that is tucked away above our garage. It is my refuge when I need to escape the loud hustle and bustle of our home. I did a deep clean of the room, added some fresh flowers and set up my diffuser. It is a serene and inviting location for me to do my meditations.

Getting started is often the hardest part of incorporating a new habit into your life. If you are interested in giving meditation a try, ask yourself what strategies would work for *you*! Would reading a book or watching a documentary on the subject get you in the right mindset? Are you the type of person who operates better in the company of others? Maybe a group class would be more up your alley. Would creating an attractive nook in your home (or garden!) encourage you to visit that space more often? Look for inspiring ways to set yourself up for success!

Ignite Your Intellect

As children, our world revolves around learning and challenging ourselves mentally. Why should we have to give this up as we get older? I am so inspired by stories of people who adopt a lifelong learning approach to living.

My father is one of these people, and I was lucky enough to live in a house where I got to observe his adventures firsthand. He is a forestry engineer, who ran a building supply store while I was growing up. In his spare time, he built airplanes in our basement. He didn't have any background in this type of work, but he figured things out! From my vantage point, the whole process looked incredibly complicated. Unbelievably, he flew all three of his homebuilt planes, (one all the way from New Brunswick to Wisconsin) and obviously lived to tell of his adventures! Yes, there were a few mishaps along the way, including landing on a taxiway instead of a runway at an international airport, and crashing a few times. The point is, he learned many new skills, challenged his brain *and* had a lot of fun while doing it!

As the responsibilities of adulthood pile on, do you ever find yourself feeling a bit stale? Does it feel like you are plodding along on the same path day in day out? Maybe it's time to up your mental game by giving your mind a boost. Challenging yourself intellectually is a great way to pull yourself out of a slump. Yes, starting from scratch with a project or skill that has a steep learning curve can often feel a bit intimidating or scary. For many of us, it's been a long time since we've taken on the role of student.

I felt this way when I decided to write my first book. It had been ages since I had done any writing in a structured format. My word processing skills were as basic as they come. Taking the plunge and just going for it really ignited a renewed sense of enthusiasm in me. I enjoyed re-connecting with writing and improving my grammar and vocabulary. Although frustrating at times, I successfully figured out the "tech" side of self-publishing, learning how to maneuver my way through the Amazon KDP self-publishing platform and setting up my social media accounts. These skills helped me feel youthful and more current! Writing has given me more confidence and a mental lift.

Is there a new skill or an area of study that has piqued your interest? Have you been putting off exploring this area because of your insecurities or a perceived lack to time? Maybe it's time to reignite your spark and set yourself up for a challenge! Once again, your wellness journal is a great place to brainstorm a list of fresh and challenging ideas. Push yourself and come up with a list of ten or twenty, and then pick the one that pops out the most from the page.

Elevating Actions and Inspiration

- Our mental and physical health are so inter-connected, it's impossible to separate the two. Elevating your overall sense of wellbeing involves adopting healthy habits that are both tangible and intangible in nature.

- Now is a great time to pull out that wellness journal. View it as a loving and patient friend, who offers a listening ear with no judgement. Take stock of where you are spending most of your time and energy in life, and get honest with yourself. Are these activities and interests still bringing you joy, or is it time to close the book and move on?

- Inspire yourself to reduce your stress levels and quiet your busy mind by exploring mindfulness. Set yourself up for success by seeking out a teacher or mentor to guide you through the process. Create a small corner in your home that can serve as a refuge and a peaceful space to connect with yourself. Seek out a motivating podcast or book on the subject of mindfulness. Tap into what gets you inspired, and start there.

- Adopt an approach to life that embraces lifelong learning. Challenge yourself intellectually to keep your mind sharp and your confidence up. Pull out that journal again and brainstorm a list of new and bold ideas that you've been holding back on.

A NOTE FROM THE AUTHOR

Thank you so much for reading my book! I genuinely hope that some of my ideas and tidbits of inspiration resonated with you. On a personal level, I have enjoyed reflecting on my own journey to elevate my health. I certainly don't have all the answers, but it is both fun and rewarding to share thoughts and open the discussion with others. We all have something to offer each other, and we all have something to learn from each other. My wish is that I have sprinkled you with a few seeds of inspiration that will grow into a lush garden of habits and behaviours that nourish your body, mind and soul.

If you enjoyed my writing, please check out my other books, *Elevate the Everyday* and *Elevate Your Personal Style*. They offer a similar flavour and are also designed to share motivational tips to bring more joy, comfort, vitality and peace into your life!

I also have a tiny have a favor to ask! I would greatly appreciate it if you would take the time to leave an honest review of my book on Amazon. Not only does this help others discover my work, but it allows me to connect with my readers and gain insight into our shared interests.

Much love,

Jennifer

ABOUT THE AUTHOR

Jennifer Melville is a self-published author. She decided to embark on a writing career because she wanted to tap into a community of like-minded individuals who share in her enthusiasm for living well and seeking ways to elevate daily life. She is a professional accountant by trade, who approaches life with an analytical and observant mind. Jennifer has been exploring the concept of elevating the everyday for over twenty years. She is passionate about family, health, fitness, fashion, nutrition, nature and all the beauty life has to offer.

Jennifer lives by the sea in beautiful Nova Scotia, Canada with her husband, two sons and little poodles Coco and Junior.

You can connect with her by email, on her blog, or on her Instagram page.

jenniferlynnmelville@gmail.com
www.theelevatedeveryday.com
www.instagram.com/the.elevated.everyday

BONUS:

50 AFFIRMATIONS TO ELEVATE YOUR HEALTH

I thought it would be fun to create a list of "quick hits" that we could all reach for when we are in need of a motivational boost. None of us is immune to slumps! These affirmations are here to lift you up and set you back on track.

1. I am motivated to act in ways today that will lead to a long life of vitality, good health and happiness.
2. I envision myself as someone who is glowing with health from the inside out.
3. My strong and fit body allows me to flow through my days with ease and energy.
4. I am someone who exudes good health. I am thriving as I age because I take care of my body.
5. I love surrounding myself with inspiring images, thoughts and people. Keeping my thoughts positive helps me stay motivated and inspired about my healthy choices.

6. Every day I focus on making choices and decisions that will make me feel elevated and healthy. I choose positivity over negativity.

7. I am my biggest cheerleader. When I feel a wave of enthusiasm wash over me, I jump at the chance to take advantage of it.

8. I am flexible and don't give up on my goals when an obstacle gets in my way. I find creative ways to keep moving forward instead of throwing my hands up in defeat.

9. There is no time like the present to start acting in ways that promote better health. I don't need to wait until next month or after the holidays are behind me. I'm starting to make health a priority this very minute.

10. I have a thirst for knowledge and a passion for learning. Educating myself on how to live a healthy lifestyle gives me the tools I need to succeed.

11. I make my health a priority each and every day. I schedule my wellness activities in my planner and feel proud when I cross them off my list.

12. I treat my body with kindness and patience when it is in need of a rest. I check in frequently with my physical self to ensure the steps I am taking are in my best interest.

13. When I am injured or ill, I allow my body the rest it needs. I don't let my ego bully me into ignoring warning signs that my body needs a bit of time off.

14. While I like to challenge myself, I also know my limits. I respect these limits and operate in a manner that keeps me safe.

15. I love pulling on my colorful tights and sparkly headband before I work out. I dress for my workouts in a way that inspires me to be successful and put in an energetic effort.

16. I don't let the cold weather cramp by style and keep me from enjoying activities I love, fresh air and sunshine. I've invested in high-quality winter wear that keeps me toasty while I get my body moving.

17. While I enjoy sticking to a set schedule and plan, I also have backup workout alternatives if things don't go as planned.

18. When I open my refrigerator door, I am inspired by the sight of all the fresh and healthy food on display. It's easy to grab a quick and nutritious snack.

19. I have my freezer stocked with healthy meals that I can pull together in a quick pinch if necessary. I'd rather eat a nutritious home-cooked meal than a greasy take-out option.

20. I take my health goals and choices on trips and vacations with me. I find ways to remain active while away from home, and do my best to eat in a healthy manner, while still enjoying treats.

21. I love reading about nutrition and educating myself on how to best feed my body for optimal health.

The more I learn, the more I am inspired to stick to my goals.

22. I love starting my day with invigorating exercise. The energy I receive from it flows through me all day long.

23. Starting my day with a healthy, nourishing breakfast is an act of self-love that I deserve.

24. I am open to trying new activities and forms of exercise. I realize I don't have to be good at something to enjoy the health benefits it has to offer.

25. While I enjoy working out with other people, I am also very motivated from within. I enjoy solo activities as well as they are easy to fit into my busy schedule.

26. I love the invigorating feeling that follows after a good workout. I don't mind the slight discomfort I feel during exercise because I know that my efforts will pay me back with better health.

27. Exercise is my friend, and I am grateful for its presence in my life. I feel fortunate to be able to participate in physical activities.

28. Exercise is not a chore. It is a gift I give myself.

29. I love having strong, toned muscles.

30. Taking the time to stretch each day leaves me feeling relaxed and peaceful.

31. I don't mind exercising in the cold. I dress warmly and feel invigorated by the sense of the crisp fresh air entering my lungs.

32. Nothing quenches my thirst better than cool, fresh water. I reach for it regularly throughout the day.

33. I seek small ways to motivate myself each day. I keep energizing songs and inspiring quotes at my fingertips, and draw on them when needed.

34. I enjoy rewarding myself with little treats each day to celebrate my success. Extra time in the shower, or a quiet moment to relax by myself feel decadent.

35. I am motivated to set a good example for my children. I know they are watching and learning about living a healthy lifestyle from me! Modelling healthy behaviours is important to me.

36. I really enjoy connecting with my friends during our group workout. It is something to look forward to while I'm sweating.

37. I love getting outdoors each day for my walk. It makes me feel alive.

38. There is nothing like a great song to get me energized. I have such an awesome workout playlist that I look forward to listening to.

39. I enjoy perusing the pages of my wellness journal. I like that I have an easy source of inspiration to pick up and reinvigorate my mindset.

40. I write down my exercise plans each day and make sure they are a priority in my schedule.

41. I love getting in my workouts in the morning and don't mind getting up a bit earlier to fit them in. They help me start my day with a clear mind and a boost of energy.

42. I make time for my daily exercise because my own happiness and health are top on my list of priorities.

43. When the weather doesn't cooperate with my plans, I view this as an opportunity to shift my focus. It feels good to change things up and keep things fresh.

44. I love the delicious feeling of a good night's rest. My calming bedtime routine and cozy bed allow me to drift off in a state of relaxation. I wake up feeling so well rested and enthusiastic about the day ahead.

45. I don't feel guilty taking naps when my body needs them. Even a short rest gives me the energy boost I need to make it through the day.

46. I look forward to holidays and celebrations and never stress about overindulging. I savour seasonal treats without going overboard (except for fresh local blueberries!)

47. I focus my time and energy on activities that are important and uplifting to me. I recognize when it is time to let go of something in my life and I don't feel guilty about it.

48. I'm committed to my meditation practice. It makes me feel more centered and better able to cope with the emotional ups and downs of life.

49. I'm always seeking out new learning opportunities to remain sharp and current. I enjoy challenging myself intellectually and the confidence boost it gives me.

50. I love myself. This allows me to make decisions that are in my best interest because I care about my own health and wellbeing.

Made in the USA
Middletown, DE
10 June 2025